radiation

days

Also by Lynn Hoffman

The Bachelor's Cat

bang BANG

Philadelphia Personal

Short Course in Beer

The New Short Course in Wine

radiation

days

the rollicking, lighthearted
story of a man and his cancer

lynn hoffman

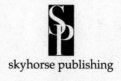

skyhorse publishing

Skyhorse Publishing books may be purchased in bulk at special discounts for sales promotion, corporate gifts, fund-raising, or educational purposes. Special editions can also be created to specifications. For details, contact the Special Sales Department, Skyhorse Publishing, 307 West 36th Street, 11th Floor, New York, NY 10018 or info@skyhorsepublishing.com.

Skyhorse® and Skyhorse Publishing® are registered trademarks of Skyhorse Publishing, Inc.®, a Delaware corporation.

Visit our website at www.skyhorsepublishing.com.

10 9 8 7 6 5 4 3 2 1

Library of Congress Cataloging-in-Publication Data is available on file.

Cover design by Glen Edelstein
Front cover photo: Thinkstock

Print ISBN: 978-1-62873-718-9
Ebook ISBN: 978-1-62914-064-3

Printed in the United States of America

For Hugh Gilmore and J

I am immensely fond of capital J
and not because
it is the first letter
in your name or because
it initiates Justice
or wanders with Jew.
I am immensely fond of capital J
for its generosity, for the way
it dips and scoops and offers up
what it spills. I love its versatility,
the way it hangs from the stern and
steers or hangs from the ceiling
and takes my coat. I like, no, love
how little it holds in its curve,
how little it cares for holding,
how blithely it lives from jewel
to jewel to jewel.

Author's Note

~ This is a comedy about coming alive, about stumbling to the light, swimming up out of the depths, and breathing again. It's about finding out what matters and letting go of the rest. Incidentally, it's also about friendship, cancer, medicine, small pleasures, lifting weights, and laughing at my own jokes. The story is told in first-person voice; that's the way I told it as it was happening. It's the voice I use to talk to friends, and this is a story you'd share with friends. I think I'll start the story for you just the way it started for me: right in the middle of things on a summer night in Philadelphia.

How I Found Out

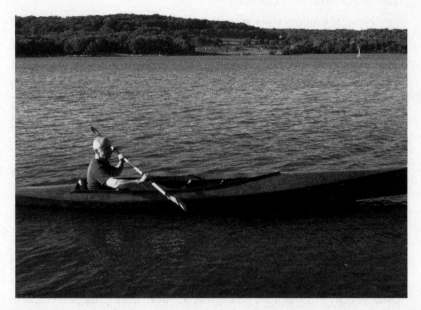

A bit down by the stern, but who wouldn't be?

⮵ The business with the allergies and aches and pains in my head wasn't getting any better, and then I woke up around 2:00 a.m. on August 7 hawking up bloody gobs from my throat. It turns out that Temple Hospital had an ear, nose, and throat specialist (ENT) on call at the emergency room and Jefferson Medical Center didn't, so we spent the night on North Broad Street. CAT scans, a chest X-ray, blood tests, nothing conclusive, but the bleeding stopped, and I got an appointment for the next Friday with a doctor in ENT (although they disdain the term ENT here; it's otolaryngology, thank you).

So, it's Friday the 13th, and J and I go for this appointment. We'll call the physician Dr. Rice-A-Roni. She checks out pretty good on the web: Johnny Hopkins, lots of publications. She slides a tube down my nose—she's the fourth or fifth doc to do this—and says, "It's cancer."

Now, if you ever want to stop the chitchat in a room and get everyone's attention, you can't do better than that. J's a doctor, and she tries a little professional optimism: Could it be an infection? Nope, cancer. Lymphatic. Cancer. Oh. Rice-A-Roni's tone wasn't exactly the chirpy one where someone tells you, "It's a girl!" but it wasn't very gentle, either—she rolled her eyes conspicuously at J's suggestion that we consult the infectious disease guy. There may have been a tiny bit of "gotcha." Anyway, shitty way to hear shitty news. It's possible that you're never going to warm up to the person who tells you that you have cancer, but I don't think anyone gets well with this lady as their doc.

So the biopsy was yesterday, and the preliminary look suggested yes, cancer, and maybe even a lot of it. Squamous cell, head and neck. Usually only smokers are so honored, but drinking helps a bit, too.

• • •

So, now we move on to discovering how many cells, how big, and how widespread. (Radiation and chemo are the usual treatment—loss of the power of speech, the sense of taste, and the ability to swallow are the usual side effects.) Next thing is the PET scan. (I'll promise no puns if you will, too.) This is a test that uses a radioactive tracer to look for disease in the body. It's part of a process called *staging*, which defines how bad it is, what your chances are, and what the doctors can do about it. That's the medical problem. The life issue is that I'm not sure what the timetable is here. Do I have a summer of sailing to look forward to, or should I not even buy green bananas? Bulletins as they break. Anyway, I'm composing a bucket list, and I'm taking suggestions. There's that sailplane ride with Peter over the autumn hills of Central Pennsylvania. I hear there's a butterfly house in British Columbia and a steak house in Tampa. I want to see if I can afford to leave enough money to keep one little corner of Fairmount Park wildlife friendly and clear of invasives. I want to be a little more Buddhist, maybe even a touch yogic. I want to taste a few things. I think I might want to record a poem or two, if I have a voice left to do it with. Definitely the porn novel, probably the missing kid story, too. I'd like to write one song. I'm surprised that there's not a lot of travel on my list so far—just being near water.

Of course, as we get down to the end, it may turn out that what I really want is two exotic dancers, a room filled with *Tastykake*s, pictures of all my dogs and cats, a Waylon Jennings album, and a set of headphones. It's not very likely, but stay tuned.

Here's what I know: I know I have a cancerous tumor growing in my throat. I know that it hurts. I know that I have a chance of surviving it after a round of radiation treatments and chemotherapy, but no one seems to know just what that chance is. I know we're all going to die, and—even though I expected my death to happen to some futurized creature who looked like me but wasn't—now I know that death happens in a very real, touchable present. Now, for instance.

I also know that my kayak, November, is ready to go in the water. Building her was a bit over my head, and any real craftsman

3

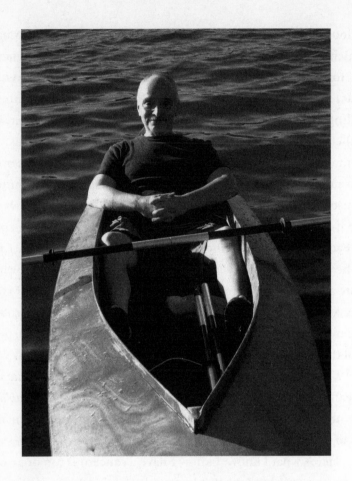

would probably snort at her, but she looks pretty good from ten feet away, and now I know that she paddles like a dream.

Tomorrow, I take in a bit of general anesthesia, and Dr. Ridge takes a close look at the tumor. I guess that the fun starts next week.

So, how do I feel? That seems to be the best question right now, partly because it's the only one I can answer. I'm not particularly scared—although I don't know why. It seems like a reasonable person would be at least a little fearful, and instead I feel calm in an emergency. Like when the wind kicks up and you're still under full sail. What I do feel is sad: I hate the thought of leaving the party early. My fantasy was that I'd see my daughter graduate from law school, maybe hold a grandchild or two.

For today, I can tell you that a little wooden boat you built yourself is a very nice thing to look at.

My Favorite Gown

∼ Fox Chase Cancer Center is no ordinary hospital. If you've been in a hospital lately, there's a good chance that you ended up thinking of yourself as, oh, *a piece of meat* or *an experimental subject* or *a case number* or even *lucky to have lived through it*. The Fox Chase people, on the other hand, seem determined to treat patients like people.

It's partly in the way they greet you, partly the pleasant sense of self-disclosure: my anesthesiologist has written a novel, my nurse is married to a pharmacist, the surgery resident loves Marques de Caceres, and so on. What really gets the message across, though, is the gown. Ever shivered through the time outside the operating room, wondering if they were planning on freezing you to stanch the bleeding? At Fox Chase, they have a gown with a paper bag inside it. It's called an Air Bear or some such. The bag has openings that look like the ones on vacuum cleaner bags, and they attach to a hose at the side of your bed. The hose brings heated or cooled air and puffs up the inner bag. It's the cozy patient process. Just to make it almost too good, the thing ties in the front! Whoever would have thought of such a thing? How can a person be cured without their bare butt being exposed to dozens of complete strangers? A nice gown. Better yet, I think I have the perfect earrings to go with it.

In fact, there's only one question that troubles me about the Fox Chase gown:

My Favorite Gown

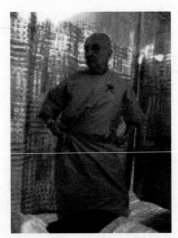

Is it too busy for daytime?

• • •

So, maybe no taste, no smell. Who will I be without them? I taught culinary arts for fifteen years. I write about the taste of wine and beer. Will there be any of me left after the taste is gone?

Subtractions

～ The biopsy's back: it's stage IV. Or is that stage 4 or stage for getting the hell out of here? Anyway, stage IV is as bad as it gets.

A consequence of radiation to the head is a loss or a distortion of the sense of taste. Food tastes too salty, too sour, like metal, or not at all. You probably won't be able to chew much anyway, so "food" in this context means a puree of something or another. You don't eat anymore; you feed. One of my doctors said something about a surgically inserted feeding tube.

So, there. In a week or two one of the sweet centers of my life will disappear. Food, making it, enjoying it, sharing it, telling stories about it, all gone. Food (and drink, too) have been my music, my art, my dance, my favorite way to connect with people.

This hasn't happened yet, so all I can do is wonder: What will I do with the passion? Is it transferable like a bank account, or is it rooted in place like a tree? There's also a darker worry:

Who will I be when the food and wine are gone?

My bet right now is that the object of passion has very little to do with it. You love what you love because you love—and then you had to pick out something to unload the love on. Not that we don't have predilections—there's not much chance I'm going to become a fan of stock-car racing or cow tipping. And I find myself thinking

Subtractions

a lot about Philly's Fairmount Park and Carpenter's Woods these days, maybe about adding them to the list of things that really matter to me. They're beautiful this time of year: false fall, crickets, asters, dayflowers, and pokeweed all over. Those woods could use a friend or two—let's see what I can do.

It's Really about Death and Time

~ What's it worth to you to live another year? How many arrows will you put up with? How often are you willing to puke? What's a good day—no, what's a good enough day? Is there anything in your life that you care about so much that you'll let the archer shoot every day rather than take Death's hand away and let him see you? How overwrought will my writing get?

So far, there is something for me. There's my kid; there's poetry and storytelling. There's the memory of teaching, eating, drinking, dancing, and being silly. There's the flight to Milan and the train to New York. There's a love; there are friends. There's curiosity, vanity, and, even still, a bit of lust, a love of laughing.

But I'm pretty thin, and the price of time gets higher with each tick. Stay tuned.

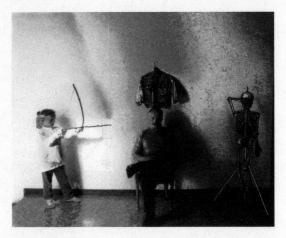

The Good Doctor—
Part One

∿ An old girlfriend hears that I'm sick and gives a call. We dated so long ago that there is mostly nostalgia in our conversations—as if we had once studied with the same irascible scholar and get to chuckle now at his failures as well as our own.

She says, "What I want to know is, do you have a really good doctor?"

This shuts me up better than the sore throat. How the hell do I know? For me to be able to tell that a doctor was good, I'd at least have to know more about the topic at hand than the doctor herself. Ideally, I should know more and have a deeper understanding of the context of the disease, too.

And I don't. I completely forgot to go to medical school—I don't even watch hospital shows on TV. In fact, I'm so puzzled by my complete naiveté in the face of such an important question that I'm starting to wonder about what I do know about doctors. How do any of us know whether any of them are any good?

One thing I could do is ask other doctors, but there's a problem. It's the same as mine, but worse. How do they know? And if they knew, would they tell? Did you ever hear a doctor say something negative about another doctor? Me neither.

One consolation: medical school and licensing procedures probably weed out most of the dingbats. But you know the old joke: what do they call the student who came in last in her class in the worst medical school in the country? You know what they call her: "doctor."

Here's all I've figured out so far: if you ask a doctor a question, you should get a complete, understandable answer. *Complete* means that all the nuances, probabilities, and uncertainties of the situation ought to be there. If the answer isn't complete enough, ask the next question: go deeper 'til you're in over your own head. If the doctor can't answer your question, you don't have a good doctor. *Understandable* means that you'd feel comfortable repeating it to someone else.

Now I place a lot of faith in this technique—probably because it's the only one I've got. Well, there's one other: you want a doctor who gives a shit. That's partly because it's nicer to be around someone like that and partly because you can assume that his caring will spur him on to know more and do his best.

So, I've knitted these two lame little threads into my only line for hooking a good doctor: my doctor, Brad Fenton, is a good doctor—a healer and a smart guy. I ask him, "Brad, if it were you, who would you go to?"

I realize that this is pretty pathetic: what I really want to know is, out of all the patients whom Dr. X has seen, how many got better and how many croaked? How does that compare with Dr. Y? My doctor says that he doesn't really know the answer, and my old girlfriend—like me—can't even begin to guess.

So, while we're at it, let me ask you—yes, you: Do you have a really good doctor? How do you know? And if you really know, would you mind coming and checking these guys out for me?

Freaking Out

 ～ The nice doctor is explaining how radiation therapy works: a gun-beam of radiation is aimed at the tumor. The radiation kills the cancer cells by messing with their DNA. Normal cells that get shot by accident (innocent bystander cells) are pretty good at replacing their DNA. The cancer cells, being more like undifferentiated stem cells and all geared up for growing, aren't very good at making DNA, so they die. Yahoo.

Of course there's a problem here for the gun-totin' cancer doc. The tumor's on the inside, and except for a few cases where they use implantable pellets, the radiation comes from the outside. How do you aim? The current answer is that you hold someone's head completely still and take a CT scan picture (the CT shows the tumor and normal cells differently). The picture is in 3D, and it acts like a map. Then the CT scanner passes it off to an X-ray machine, which shoots where the map tells it to.

Here's the trick: in order for the map to help the X-ray beam, the person's head has to be in the same place every time. Otherwise the radiologist is just a touch-typist who doesn't know which keys to start from. He's shooting fish in a barrel in the dark. And so on. So, to make sure the beam's hitting what the scan is saying, your head has to be in exactly the same place every time.

Here's how they do that. They make a mesh mask of your head. The mask has to be very tightly fitted to your face. Then they frame the mask with a flange and bolt it, with your head inside it, down to the CAT scan table. Then they take your picture, move you and the mask over to the X-ray table, bolt you down again, and fire away. From then on, every time you come for radiation therapy, you're in register and that ol' tumor is right in their sights.

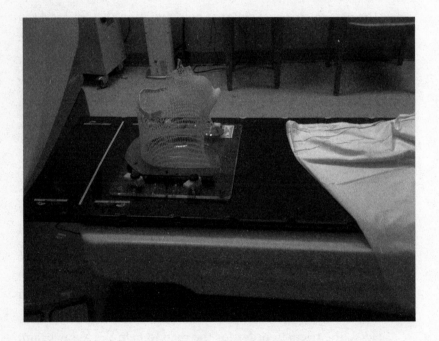

I guess the resemblance to the lethal injection table is coincidental. The mask is the mesh contraption. Look at it. Can you feel your head held immobile on the table and the mesh tight against your skin?

It's at about this time in the explanation that I started to think, *You're going to bolt me down with my head in a what?* As soon as the vision of that confinement started to form, I could feel my heart start to race. Fear, no, *panic*—sheer animal, get-me-the-hell-outta-here panic—took over. I find myself wondering what death from this cancer would be like. Gotta be better than the mask. I'm giving thinking too much credit here. There's no thought involved at all. There's just a very short loop that goes from the image of being bolted (bolted!) down by my head to wild, pulse-throbbing, muscle-twitching, sweat-panic. All flight, no fight. This ain't happening. Not to this citizen.

Later, minutes later, the thinking sets in. I remember seeing death masks of this person or that—folks who were important enough to be memorialized and who had no say in the matter anyway. *Saints in white plaster*, I sing to myself, ripping off the Moody Blues tune, something about *reaching the end*. My kid, my books in progress, the sweetness of autumn, the beauty of J, Garth Stein novels, another baseball season, paddling the Pine Barrens. Shit. The ticket to life has to be bought with this? OK, I'll take it like a man. I ask the doctor the big, manly question, say the thing that would make my daughter proud. Is there a drug for that?

Is There a Drug for That?

~ There's a conversation the day before the radiation simulation. Mine is with Dr. Galloway, a young, pleasant man with a gentle way about him. I tell him that I'm in absolute horror of what he has in mind for me, and I want to know if he has any drugs for the Mortal-Fear-of-Being-Confined Syndrome.

I don't want you to think that drugs were my first resort. Oh, no. First I tried mindfulness—breathing exercises to see if I could substitute reality for the fantasies that ran screaming around inside my head. Not a chance. Thinking about the mask beat paying attention to the breath every time. Then I gave myself a guided image. I imagined Maitreya dancing backward through the future to the Pure Land, where he does a soft-shoe number with the Amida Buddha to the tune of "Tea for Two." About the time I got to "me for you, and you-oo-oo for me," I saw them both imprisoned in plastic mesh and crushed, with little Buddha oozes coming out between the threads. Not good, not medicinal, heart rate hitting about 120.

So, my question to Dr. Galloway is simple, heartfelt, and almost completely without shame:

"Got any drugs for that?"

He does. In fact, he whirls immediately in his swivel stool to fetch his prescription pad, almost as if he had been waiting for me to ask. The little pill is five milligrams of Xanax. Lots of people have problems with the mask, he assures me. He orders me one for every day of treatment—a nice touch, since it gives me a gauge with which to watch the Roentgens go by. Out of pills? Well, then, you must be done with radiation.

I took one pill before J and I left the house. An hour later, in the waiting area, I'm hearing my heart beat and wondering if I can dig a tunnel right the hell out of here. J assures me that my dose, a half a milligram, ain't much, so I took another point-fiver—the one that I brought along just in case. I may have messed the metric up a little here: at two tabs per bolting down, I'll go through this bottle at the halfway point. I'm sick about mucking up the meter—but I'll bet there's a drug for that, too.

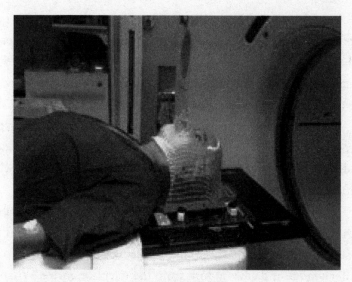

How would you feel?

The Passing of a Pronoun, or What Happened to "My"?

∼ Someplace early in the cancer countdown, the possessive pronoun, first-person singular starts to sound sort of silly. "My"? My what? What could possibly still be mine? Or, maybe, how weird is it to maintain that you can own anything when the *you* who does the owning might disappear at any minute? Can a puff of smoke take out a mortgage? Do waves have driver's licenses? It becomes suddenly very easy to look out and see things you own dancing on their merry way without you. My dog, my car, my books, my house.

Maybe it's still OK to talk about my books (the ones I wrote), my friends, my students, my kid, my karma. Maybe. Chances are that the link with the dogs—all of them—is eternal. Of course, Spike the cat is mine forever and vice-versa. (I could call them all now, and maybe we'll huddle together under a blanket and refuse to come out.)

Even allowing for these exceptions, owning something starts to sound not impossible, but at least deluded, and at worst obscene. And once the principle of the thing becomes evident, the whole foundation of "my" starts to look pretty shaky.

I guess that if "my" starts to disappear, "me" either disappears with it, or it's all that's left. When I think about that for a bit, I find myself starting to laugh, sort of like the crow who flies just out of the hunter's range and caws at him from the telephone wire. Whatever

18

goes on, nothing can happen to "me," and we're all fine, purring and snorting and barking together in a nice warm bed.

• • •

So far, "having cancer" has been mostly about dealing with bad news. This week, it's turned into palpable disease. Every day, I have a little more pain in my throat and head, and I get a bit weaker. I lose a little weight, and my throat closes a bit more. I go to the gym, and I leave because I'm tired, not because I'm finished. There are other symptoms, too. I would like to start treatment now.

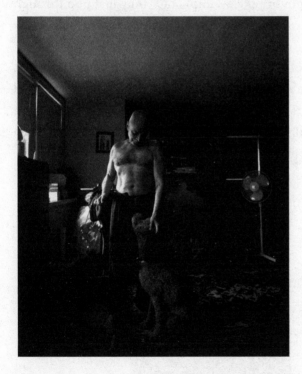

Before treatment:
162 pounds,
twenty-five pushups,
one dog

Tuesday, they install a chemotherapy port—a little vein valve that lets the chemo in and the blood out. Then, maybe later this week . . .

• • •

Send in the Cheems

Back in the bad old days, every time a patient got chemotherapy, they opened up a fresh vein. Between the finite number of veins and the apparently infinite number of occasions for opening them, a crisis emerged. Not only were they running out of veins, but some of the repeat offenders were inclined to infection.

So the solution is the port—something like a gas cap semi-permanently inserted into your blood supply. There's a cap and a valve that leads to a tube into a vein. Whenever they need to pump something in or take a sample out, they just pop through the thin skin that now covers the valve and add or subtract as they wish.

Getting one of these installed is painless, and they tell me it takes about fifteen minutes. The procedure is done by a pro called an interventional radiologist. I take this to mean that he's a surgeon with instrument flight rules training or a radiologist who just hated all the fun he was missing.

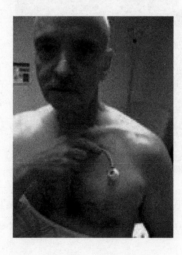

The Passing of a Pronoun, or What Happened to "My"?

You wait for your port placement in a state called NPO, or *nil per os*—nuttin' in the mouth. They say it has something to do with keeping your gut free, but any anthropologist would recognize it as part of the separation phase of an initiation ritual. I understand that at Sloan-Kettering, they make you sit in a smoky sweat lodge for two hours, and at Johns Hopkins they have something called "Beat them to starboard, then stick in the port." So, I guess it could be worse.

Here at Fox Chase, after your port is implanted, you have about an hour to get a mushy sandwich past your jaws, and then you go to the chemo lounge. The lounge is a set of screenable areas with a big easy chair for the guest of honor (at last, your own BarcaLounger!), a guest chair, a TV, a reading light, and a pump on a stand.

They hang some bags on the pump stand, connect them to a tube coming out of your brand-new port, wish you luck, and walk away while they drip-drip-drip you: 2.5 liters of saline, plus the drug itself. You read, you doze, you get up eleven times to pee (*hydration* is the big word here). You're slightly, pleasantly out of it.

My friend Laura drove me there in the morning and picked me afterward. (There's no way you could drive home safely: too woozy, almost post-physical. I might try a triple-axel on Germantown Avenue.) She also helped me pop a few wheelies in the wheelchair going out the door.

The amazing thing is that the pain that I've been living with was reduced by 90 percent with no pain meds involved. They tell me that's typical. Side effects? Well, I slept twelve hours last night (listened to the seventh- and eighth-inning Phillies beating the Braves and then nodded out) and may go sleep some more now.

Had a little twinge of nausea. All in all, I'd say it's a pretty good trade-off. Now, if only this stuff cured cancer . . .

• • •

21

The Odds Go Up

There are two kinds of tumors that form where mine is. One is the squamous or scaly-cell tumor. It's caused mostly by smoking and drinking, and it's about 50 percent curable. The other kind is caused by human papillomavirus (HPV), and it's about 80 percent curable. There have been chances for a month to find out which cause was behind my effect, but Dr. Murphy and his Law delayed the news a bit.

No matter now. It's an HPV tumor—here's a picture of its author:

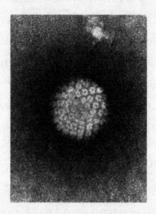

Charming fellow. I'd like to have one as a pet if only I didn't already have a whole family of them. Maybe I'll settle for a plush animal version. I'll say more about HPV later, but one intriguing note is that this is about the only cancer-causing organism against which there is a vaccine. Yup. A vaccine. They're giving it only to kids these days—and mostly to girls—but a lot of cancers—including mine—could have been prevented with the shot.

Maybe someday we'll chat about how some health officials and conservative legislators object to giving the vaccine for moral reasons (moral reasons!), but not now. Eighty percent feels like quite an improvement, and I think I'll enjoy that feeling.

• • •

Crash!

My friend Hugh Gilmore drives me on Thursday to my first radiation session. I've already had chemo number one, and while he's driving, I'm extrapolating. "If I feel this much better on day one, it's probably going to be all right." Hugh and I make a date for some serious porch-sitting and world-repairing tomorrow, Friday. Nice way to start the weekend, eh? On the Road to Recovery, cancer cells quivering with fear as my little friends the electrons start swatting them around. Yeah, maybe we'll even sing a bit.

That Friday afternoon, a few hours after the second radiation treatment, the brick wall comes crashing down. I'm riding home with Charlie, my co-op driver. Charlie's been down the cancer trail himself, and he's mildly, quietly positive. The third day's the worst, he says. It wasn't fun, but he beat it. I've got a little positive glow going myself. The pain has lessened—no more pencils stabbing in the ear canal, no tender boils in my throat. Then, just about the time the car pulls to the curb in front of J's house, I'm sure that there's no way I can get out of the car, lift myself to vertical, and walk. I'm dizzy, sort of like being drunk but without the tiniest bit of fun. I do not yell, "Yahoo!" as I spiraled to the ground. Nor did I wish anybody a Happy New Year. I'm nauseated, too. There's a golf-ball-size chunk of something in my throat that's trying to kick its way out. My fingers seem to work, but nothing else does. I try to explain my predicament, but nothing comes out. I don't remember how I got inside—the expression "doubled over" comes to mind. Images from Dante pop up: Paolo and Francesca puff by, or the souls of the damned eager to hit the ferry to Staten Island. I notice that most of the anti-nausea meds are sedatives of one sort or another. That seems like a good idea, and I sleep. I think Hugh called sometime in there to check up on me, but I can't remember what I said, and I'm hoping he doesn't. It's now about a full day later. I'm going to see if I can stand up.

• • •

Hospitalized

Yesterday as I was getting ready to head out for radiation day number three, Friday's dizziness came back, and I blacked out. Not the two-and-a-half-bottle-of-wine, danced-all-night kind of blackout, more like a little swirly gray down that leaves you staring up at the bathroom ceiling with a certain pale sense that something's horribly wrong and you probably have a checkerboard bathroom tile pattern embedded on your cheek. Somehow I called J. She suggested trying to get downstairs to unlock the door so that whoever came to get me wouldn't need to break it down. Somehow I called Hugh and he came and dumped my semiconscious ass into the car. So I checked into the hospital at Fox Chase where I'm getting my treatment. It turns out that I was dehydrated. The chemo-chemical from chemo number one was drying me out so much that body systems were shutting down. I got to the point where I wasn't thirsty—or hungry—and was a little nauseated, so I drank less water and didn't eat much and . . .

So, anyway, the deal is that the doctors try to kill the cancer, and the stuff they use tries to kill you. The stuff is not smart enough to tell the difference between cancer and you, so it kills you a little, too. So then the docs give you stuff to ameliorate the effect of the cancer-killing stuff. This stuff is only slightly smarter than the first bunch, so while it helps a bit, it has some drawbacks of its own, which need correction. And then there's another drug, and so on. Yesterday's drying out was just one body system overwhelmed. In the time it takes them to get the numbers right for all the different systems, you get your ass smacked around a little. Yesterday and today I was in Fox Chase hooked up nonstop to IV saline solution. (I'm told that 0.9 percent salt water is the body's drink of choice—although you coulda fooled me.) Six or seven liters later, I'm human again, I've got a new medicine schedule, and I'm thinking of getting that bathroom floor upholstered.

What's dehydration like? I can't really tell you, but I can guess. You can't trust my report completely because one of dehydration's effects is that your brain is flooded with Vitamin Stupid. I couldn't find things that were in their usual spots; I was barely aware of anything going on around me. Did I already take that pill? Should I take another? Meditating was easy; thinking was hard. Right now, I don't remember much of what happened. I suspect that if you died from dehydration, you might not notice that you were gone.*

Back to Fox Chase tomorrow for radio day number five. And how are you?

• • •

Bolted Down—Radiation Day Number Six

It turns out that being bolted to the table isn't much worse than being screwed on the desk or nailed on the carpet. It lasts only a few minutes, and there's not much pain involved. The people at the clinic are a kind of embodied medicine: healing oozes out of them, and gets all over you. I think a daily dose of Lucille Williams, the angel at the reception desk, might cure a person of something, or at least chase away the horrors.

---

* Of course, it's always possible that there is no difference, but that line of thinking leads to a heavy sense of adolescent pessimism and some very strange sci-fi movies.

So, by radiation day number six, I'm skipping the pill. My friend J. R. Lankford gives me some quick meditation advice, and I slouch down into Meshmask-Land and feel my breath going in and out. (I'm a little embarrassed that my own Buddha nature didn't get me to this, but that's why they invented drugs.) In a few minutes it's over, and as long as I don't feel choked by the little tumor bump on the back of my tongue, it's pretty easy. I know it's silly to feel triumphant about something like being able to skip a tranquilizer, so I'll just feel lucky.

· · ·

Reluctantly Speaking—Radiation Day Number Seven

My friend Bonnie† is a farmer. She makes her way through the world with an appealing, jovial, sarcastic, cocktail-lounge tone of voice. It's not my native language, but I speak it, and she's my friend, so when she's around, I speak it with her. She visited me one day last week in the company of some other folks, and we poked and scoffed at each other for a bit. Then when we were alone, looking around to make sure nobody heard her talkin' nice, she said, "But how are you? Really."

"Today's a pretty good day," I told her, "although my voice is sounding weird. Does it sound strange to you?"

"Well, you do sound different. Not so hyper—though you're not really hyper, exactly." She took a few seconds' pause. "But, um, not as aggressive as usual, but then you're not really aggressive, either.

---

† In order to preserve Bonnie's reputation as a tough gal I've changed her name in this piece.

But it's different." For a second there, the look on her face could have been taken for affection.

It took me a while, but I think I understand what Bonnie was saying.

It hurts a little when I talk, and the longer I talk, the more it hurts. So I'm a little less generous with the words. I try to let them out in a low-pressure, easy-on-the-throat, breathy rhythm. If someone talks over me, I just shut up. I never repeat myself anymore. If you ask me what I just said, I wait quietly until your brain catches up to your ears—invariably, it does.

I can't imagine what this new voice must sound like to other people—it's certainly not the same changed voice that I'm hearing. I hope it doesn't sound calculated, and I really pray that it doesn't sound wise.

What I take it to be is that now that the price of words has gone up, I have to be more frugal. I'd hate to be stingy, but I never heard of anybody's expression that was damaged by a little sparseness, by a dash of economy, or by a bit of restraint. Brevity's not in the nature of my Irish side—there are no haiku in Gaelic, don't ya know—but a man grows up even as a man grows old.

I remember being advised that an artist should change his name every ten years to keep from being trapped in the cage of his latest work. Maybe changing your voice once every major disease or so would have the same effect. I don't know what to make of it.

Stay tuned.

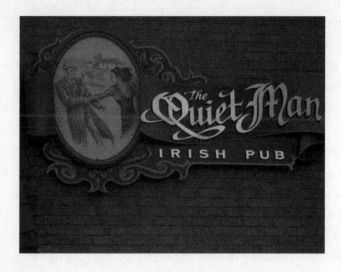

• • •

These days I'm staying in Mt. Airy—that's a neighborhood in Philadelphia. I'm in a stone house that's about one hundred feet from Carpenter's Woods. The stone is spangly schist, and the outside sparkles in the sun. On the inside, there's not much sparkle: small windows, low ceilings, lots of dark surfaces. I don't really live in this house; I sort of ride it like a fly on a melon, sticking to my little sliver of bed, my small pile of books, my square of couch.

It's a good house for writing, a bad house for wasting time. Today I wondered if I would die here, maybe lying on my side facing a blond wood night stand. I can't really picture it, and I decide that it doesn't matter much.

The Big Picture in Two Parts

Part One

Here's what I'm looking at: there's thirty-five days of radiation therapy and three bouts of chemotherapy. Chemotherapy's friends would call it "chemo"—but now that you mention it, chemo doesn't have any friends outside the companies that sell the stuff.

Today was radiation dose number nine. The radiation sessions happen Monday through Friday—five days a week for seven weeks. A session consists of them doing a CAT scan to make sure they are picking up where they left off, then there's about five minutes of X-ray bombardment. The whole thing takes about twenty minutes, and—in my case—happens every day exactly at noon. I've already had one chemo and told you about it; the second one is next week. The whole thing ends November 10.

When it's all over, they wait four weeks and do a CAT scan: December 8.

The scan is our report card, theirs and mine. There are three possible outcomes.

They may have killed the thing. If they have, we have a "Borrowed Time Starts Today" party. And we start looking at sailboat ads.

Or maybe they got most of it. Then they have to make a new treatment plan, and this story gets an extension. Frankly, I could do without this one.

The third possibility is that the treatment flat-out didn't work. That's the one where we have a farewell tour, sort of like the Doobie Brothers in '83 or The Band's *The Last Waltz* in '76. That was the concert where they got a big horn section behind them. Did you ever hear a more moving rendition of "Stage Fright"? You can almost feel the kernel of doubt and fear behind the public persona of the performer, and you have to be reminded that we're all performers.

And then there's the anthemic quality of "The Night They Drove Old Dixie Down," evoking . . . ah, but I digress. The third possibility is that I'm going to die soon and miss the chance to play out a weird old age. The thought still makes me more sad than scared, but mostly it makes me want accomplishment, experience, states of being, the sheer freakiness of being outdoors.

Right now, I'm working with the first outcome, the one we'll call "Thirty-Five and Out."

Part Two

Tomorrow I'm going to make crème brûlée. There's not much to making it: I'll take a cup of half and half and beat an egg into it. I'll add some sugar—maybe a tablespoon, which is a whole lot less than most folks like, but this is my food. Then I'll add some Madagascar vanilla and a few drops of dark rum.

The mix will be poured into two white ramekins; the ramekins go into a loaf pan, and I'll pour hot water around them 'til it's halfway up the side. The kitchen will have a high sharp smell—like edible air—as I put the whole bit into a 300°F oven. In about an hour, I'll take them out and let them cool, maybe even chill them a little to tighten them up. (It works on me; ought to work on pudding, too.) Then I'll sprinkle the tops with a coating of raw sugar, haul up the propane torch from the basement, and work the flame over the sugar top. There's a craft to it, of course. If I'm careful, the sugar will melt but not scorch and the room will smell of caramel. Say the name *car-a-mel*. Don't cheat on a single syllable: caramel. Sugar all grown up and ready to go out dancing.

I'll put a piece of plastic wrap over one of the dishes and put it in the reach-in. It will be a gift. Then I'll sit the other one on the counter where the skylight is rich and cool and shadowless. I'll take a teaspoon and tap the back of it on . . . what? Yes, the caramel, and it will crack. I'll make a dozen pieces or so. I'll look at them, study them like they were a map of a place I plan to visit next week. I'll smile at the vanilla-rum scent that comes through the borderlines. Then I'll dip the spoon into one of the cracks and lever up—a township? A county? Some little division of Caramel-Land. There will be exactly the right amount of eggy, dense custard clinging to the crust. I'll look for a little translucency on the edges—do you remember that TV show, *I Love Translucency*?

It will take a long time for each bit to dissolve and coat my mouth. Texture, flavor, evocation, drama. The custard will play the part of Love, and the caramel will appear in the role of Wit. I will rumble with the beauty of it; I will think of absent friends—and that, my dears, is the only possibility.

Questions from the Mask

I'm almost sorry to come back to the business about the mask and being bolted to the table and all that, but under my circumstance, it's really hard to avoid it.

For one thing, if you sleep ten hours, wake up, go get bolted down, then come home and go to sleep for another three, bolting starts to look like the high point of your day. Or at least the pimple on an otherwise flat-assed dermis of a day.

It's also true that coping with the trapped feeling of the mesh mask involves something like meditation. You know, deep relaxation, concentrate on the breath, don't anticipate, don't remember. Be here. Now, dammit.

And whether you like it or not, that's a state that lets the darndest things pop into your head. Maybe it's creativity, or maybe it's just a side effect of the constipation that comes from all those drugs. In either case, there are these things that pop into your head—the things that the experienced meditator escorts immediately out of the room and that the trapped X-ray patient hangs on to.

Here's one that came up for me: I'm signed up for thirty-five of these sessions—five times a week for seven weeks. But if I need thirty-five zaps (Why not thirty-two or thirty-eight? Did somebody do the numbers?), wouldn't it be more humane to just go seven days a week and get this business over in five weeks?

Why draw it out? Is it to give the tumor a sporting chance? Does the patient need a break? Was there a test of continuous versus interrupted radiation? Did the interrupted approach do a better job?

It turns out that the reason you don't get life-saving radiation on Saturday and Sunday is that the hospital isn't open. You don't get it 'cause they don't give it. I hope it's not just a question of doctors not wanting to work on the weekends. Does anybody know?

These days, one of the obstacles to America's having a sane health-care system is that our costs are the highest in the world. And when you're bolted down for a while, you start to wonder whether this gigantic, hideously expensive machine ought to be sitting idle for two days out of seven. And whether "we don't want to stay open on the weekend" is a good enough reason.

Bad Day/No Comment

Radiation day number fourteen is a Tuesday, and it's the worst day I've had so far. I have no energy or appetite. My sense of humor has lost its sense of direction and can't find its way home; my zest for life has been sprinkled on top of risotto and served at someone else's table. I make some rice pudding to try to fatten myself up; it is disgusting: sort of like wood chips, but not as tasty. I haven't heard from my kid or from much of my digestive tract—two contacts I've come to depend on for a sense of well-being. This is not to say that everything is going badly. Oh, no. J still shows every sign of loving me, and my friends check in regularly. ("Visualize naked women fishing," my friend Peter writes. Fly or spinning? I wonder.) My dog is dogness herself, and I swear she's working on a cure in her spare time. In fact, if I were to balance it all out, I'm sure it would all balance out. The problem is that the balance is broken: none of the good things matter much today. I have my depression armor on, and it's proving undisprovable.

Not only that, but I somehow messed up the appointment with the shrink at Fox Chase, so the chemical cavalry is probably not going to be on the way anytime soon. And, please, if you have some cheerful anodyne for me right now, check to see if I can smoke it or swallow it before you send it along.

• • •

I've been following the story of the Chilean miners who were trapped in the San Jose Mine below the Atacama Desert, although "following" is probably the wrong word for the spooky identification I feel. It's not just a matter of feeling like I'm part of the group to be rescued. (That would be too simple for my readers—cancer patient = trapped miner. You guys deserve better than that.) No, I've identified with the miners and their families and the little tent town that's grown up on the surface. I'm standing bravely with the whole country and especially Mining Minister Laurence Golborne. It makes me smile to think that I even know the name of the mining minister of Chile—I couldn't tell you the name of his counterpart here in the US.

I guess the strangest thing of all is that I've fantasized a whole community of other Chilean mine worker devotees. I imagine a worldwide group of people—tender hearts, blotting paper imaginations, maybe a little claustrophobic—small-family people who want lots of kin.

So, later tonight, when they winch Florencio Avalos to the surface, I'll be watching on the hospital TV set, and I suspect I'll cry. And to all of you who will be crying with me, I just want to say, "It's been great; we're free. I'll miss you. Goodbye."

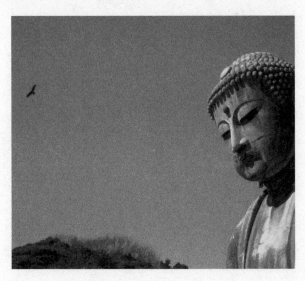

• • •

RADIATION DAYS

Coloring with the Big Box/Fox Chase

along the infusion bays
numbered Rusty Raspberry chairs, unnumbered bravelette smiles
sunken chests, ruined taste buds, traitor noses
Skanky Lime gowns
the rainbow is in the sudden,
end-of-life resolve that what matters now
is not what mattered just an Opaque Opinion ago
before we were wrapped in heated blankets
and watched the waters drip in our veins
and marveled at the waters rushing out.
before we forgave ourselves and them
and rushed to color in Goodly Green between the lines.
before the only seasoning we could stand was the Slightly Silver
clove-of-garlic moon above the trees that stand
outside the Pale Male windows of the infusion bays
where we infuse ourselves back into the world
and give Thanks Vermillion for the healing.

The Good Doctor—
Part Two

~ The other thing you really, really want to know is whether you're going to make it or not. This isn't just casual interest; it's the deal. Now, nobody on Earth expects a doctor to look you over and say, "2.7 years, maybe 2.8," but you'd think after seeing a zillion or so patients, a doctor would have a pretty good idea.

If that's true, and in fact watching hundreds of people struggle with this disease and watching some of them win and go off dancing on the beach and others lose and go off by ambulance to the hospice ... if that gives you some idea about a person's chances, none of these guys are going to tell you what they think. When you ask, they say, "Well, everybody's different." You probably knew that, and if you pursue and say, "What do you think the probabilities are?" they say something really stupid, like, "You're a person, not a probability." Actually, I knew that, too, even though I can barely croak out the question.

These brilliant folks, with ten to twelve years of training, who probably took calculus as undergrads, all of a sudden don't know what a probability is. They read papers reporting research using these very terms, and they come up blank. Try again: "What's a 50 percent confidence interval for a guy my age with this particular condition?" They still don't know what you mean. One doc at Temple Hospital even said to his younger colleague, "I forbid you to answer that question."

RADIATION DAYS

Any doctors out there? You wanna tell us what's going on here? Thanks, and there's an excellent chance, in fact a 0.99 probability, that all of us will appreciate it.

• • •

The button taped to my chest says HEAL. My friend Ashley passed it on to me by way of an exhibit about women who had been brutalized in Mexican drug wars.

Whenever I wear it, I think about Ashley and those women, and I think that it says HEAL but it really reminds me to BE GRATEFUL, because compared to those women, I'm barely hurt.

Anyway, those are just some of my pills. Aren't you glad that I'm not going to tell you what they're for?

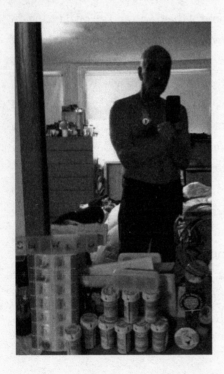

160 pounds, fifteen pushups,
lots of pills

Tumor Down, Lynn Holding Steady

∼ According to Dr. Galloway's calibrated fingertips, my tumor has shrunk to less than 40 percent of its original size. That makes it about half a centimeter in diameter. Dr. Skarbnik confirms in his soft Brazilian accent that the sucker is on the run. They both smile as they say it.

Neither one of them is willing to suggest that we might be able to stop the radiation early, though. Maybe I'll try to bargain for a chemo-reduction.

Return of the Voice

∿ Last night during the Phillies' game, I got an email saying that poems number twenty-nine and thirty have been accepted for publication in *The Centrifugal Eye*. I started writing poetry about a year ago. It was nice to find another way to get heard, but I thought of it as a substitute for fiction, not speech.

Here's poem number twenty-nine:

the grasshopper in october

he hears the tremble of the ants below
as he wakes, mulled in cold that lasted past the night
they're down there hoarding life to last beyond the snow,
he sees the crystals in the thin autumnal light

Note that the grasshopper is not complaining. No word on what the crystals are—his, theirs, everyone's.

Coincidental with this publication, my voice seems to be coming back. Last night I called family in Mississippi and managed conversation—even threw in some unnecessary words, made a joke or two. When my friend Peter came down from State College to visit, we sat and talked—chat, gossip, idle speculation—all splendidly unnecessary. OK, it's not the booming, stentorian foghorn that marks me as an American, no matter what language I'm speaking. It's not even a decent cab-hailer. But I can speak a graf if anyone's listening, and it only hurts a little.

Unless there's a surprise in store, I can forget the romantic image of the croaking mute poet, and I'll have to think of something else to scare the kids on Halloween.

Halfway Flinching/
Unflinching

∽ There was a photographer once named Ralph Eugene Meatyard. He did a lot of spooky-funny, thumb-in-your-eye photographs. Toward the end of his life—he died of cancer at forty-seven‡—he chronicled his own deterioration. The word the critics used a lot was "unflinching."

I've been doing some self-portraits recently, and I have to admit to a bit of queasiness. The body I'm photographing is old, and it's now kind of scrawny and ravaged. Why am I putting it out in the world—even forcing it under people's noses?

I remember reading an article about a Philly guy named Jerry Blavat. Jerry is one of those livin' large guys who had a lot of fun with rock and roll, shot his car a couple of times, and still keeps a job. I admire Jerry. What puzzled me was the photo—it showed sixty-seven-year-old Jerry stripped to the waist. Is this the new normalization of old age, or have we just lost some sense of when it's time to cover up for publication? The truth is, I don't know. I do know that when an aged Joe Louis was asked to strip down to boxing trunks for a Bert Stern photo, he refused, and the resultant picture—gnarled brown fists coming out of a camelhair overcoat—was a better statement about the strength of old age than the photographer's original idea.

---

‡ The same age as Kerouac when he died.

42

Halfway Flinching/Unflinching

So, what am I doing here? I'm not particularly embarrassed by my wreckage, but I'm afraid to be embarrassed by bad judgment, by getting the culture of cool completely wrong, by being overly revealing. TMI and all that. I'm thinking it might be time to flinch.

And, as soon as I say it, I know it's not time to flinch, not yet. This is what cancer looks like today, October 16, 2010.

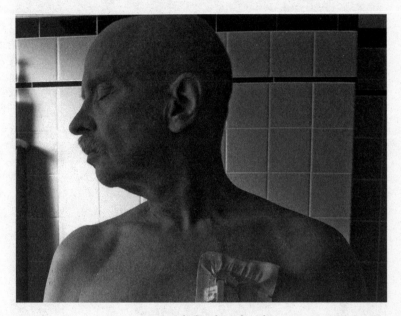

156 pounds, bright red neck

Just before I started treatment, I had a lean body mass measurement done at the gym. There was 153 pounds of skinny me and about 25 pounds of fat. Today, halfway through, at 156 total, I've got about enough fat to fry three eggs.

• • •

RADIATION DAYS

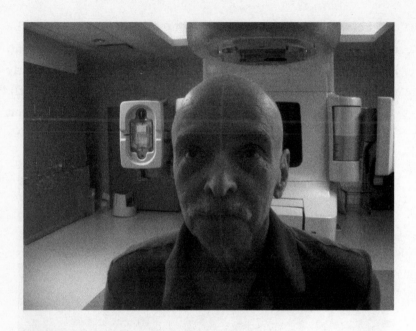

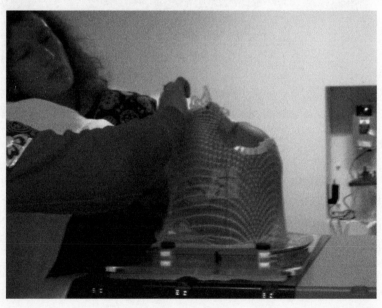

Halfway Flinching/Unflinching

cancer in january

this malignant day is the testament of our permanent place
on a frozen earth—no shoots to beg, insist, demand
on sunlight, no leaf or tree to die.
today it's cancer, swallow the stone.

it is a forever day as etched in ice as your families,
your loves, your best ideas, your many selves
the very cold is very proof.
the numbness is your promise of always-be.

what would you do if you knew
that sun would be higher in its course today
and then tomorrow and the next?

could you imagine the thaw?
what is it that lives through the death of ice?

(Published in *Forward Magazine*, 2012)

• • •

What Gets Me There

Every morning at about 11:30, I climb into my Acme Re-insifrinator. It's the new model, the one with iHeal built in. I press a few buttons, double-check it with my iPhone, and then hit SEND.

About twelve minutes later, my molecules have been reassembled in the basement of the Fahrquar Building at Fox Chase, and the radiation begins.

Not really.

What actually happens is that every midday I have to be driven to Fox Chase and then fetched back home again. I tried driving myself once—it was a big mistake, and…well, let's all be grateful that noon is not a time when there's a lot of school buses on the road.

So, every morning someone has to drive me there, wait around, and bring me back. It's an hour and a half investment on a good day. On a bad day it can be five or six. As a cab ride it's half a c-note plus, so mostly I depend on the kindness of my friends.

J is my most frequent driver, and she is burning up her vacation days catering to me and my cancer. I'll tell you more about her later. The next guy is my friend Hugh Gilmore. Hugh is a writer (*Malcolm's Wine*), book collector, storyteller, and amazing photographer who throws away more picture-genius in a day than most people enjoy in a lifetime.

The thing about Gilmore's generosity is that he barely lets you notice that it's there. Something almost makes me think that I'm doing him the favor and not the other way 'round. This is a gift. I covet that ability, but I barely have it, and I don't see it that often in others.

Two or three times a week I get to spend some nice conversational time with Hugh Gilmore, and the gift of his talk is right up there with the gift of getting my ass to radiation every day. Of course I am touched, and I almost wonder if I should be grateful to the cancer for letting me lean on my friends. Maybe not, you say? OK, but it's still a damn close thing. What I feel is enormously, mushily grateful for what gets me there. Be honest: doesn't it kinda get you there, too?

• • •

Broken Records

I've been going on for a while now about my frustration. It seems that it's impossible to find out what cancer treatments work, how they ought to be administered, and what one's chances are of living through the whole damn thing. I've been blaming the doctors, which is partially right (they should at least have a hunch). What I've been missing out on is that in a really fundamental way, no one knows what survival rates are.

We don't know because there are no uniform records kept. Right. Nobody lists the 3.2 million cases of this or that and then follows up to see what happened. Why not? Because insurance companies have lobbied against uniform records. Why? Well, suppose you knew that hospital A had a 90 percent survival rate and B had a 70 percent rate. You and every other citizen would be over at A, and B would be closed or at least in big trouble. Lotsa docs outta work there, and we can't have that, can we?

But, wait, there's more. If we could compare outcomes—could see that treatment Z is better than treatment Y—then we wouldn't buy insurance that didn't cover Z. And the insurance company that offered/covered only Y would have to cut rates or pay for better treatment. In short, my dear ones, the insurance companies don't want you to know how good your hospital is, and they surely don't want you to know how lethal your insurance might be. Comprehensive medical records—and the research they would generate—could result in everybody getting the best treatment available, but it's not in the insurers' best interests.

Is there any solution to the problem? Stay tuned.

• • •

Indignity Number Twelve—The Feeding Tube

Dignity comes from the Latin *dignitas*—a word indicating that something is worthy of respect, both honored and honorable. One of cancer's many charms is that it pretty quickly chips away at the foundations of dignity. All your assumptions about your body as inviolable and about your person being your own just don't hold anymore. You are now a battlefield for a particularly ugly kind of war between tumors and chemists, and, frankly, my dear, neither side gives a rat's ass about you.

So, you are invaded, bombarded, poked, sampled, and trampled. Here's the latest: food is so disgusting to me these days that I can barely eat. I've gone from 170 pounds to 153 (78 to 69 kilograms).

On top of that, my mouth is so dry that anything that goes in it feels like dust. I'm losing weight at about a pound a day. Now, normally, neither Bonaparte nor Wellington cares, but it turns out that my losing weight means that I'm living off myself. At first it was my own fat, but I'm out of fat now, so it's a diet of lean me. The reason this matters is that all that yummy Lynn-protein could give a false reading of kidney health, which could lead to an overdose of platinum (platinum!) in my next chemo.

Now, of course, no respectable invading army would let that happen, so before my skin folds start flapping in the breeze, General Wellingparte has a plan. His plan is to insert a feeding tube in my chest that pokes a hole in my stomach and to use that to pump food into me.

Forgive my delicacy here, but I'm horrified. You're going to stick a hose in me. I don't think so. Naturally, I have the final say, but they do have a point. Former students of mine who have listened to my stove-side rants about good food will be happy to hear that I now decide my menu based on caloric density, and my favorite flavor is milk chocolate.

• • •

Halfway Flinching/Unflinching

After a day of living with the thought (which is not exactly the same as thinking), I decide that I won't have the feeding tube, no matter what the consequences of that refusal might be. "Decide" isn't the right word, either; it makes me sound a lot more rational than I am. I just can't see me there. I tell the oncologist, Barbara Burtness. She asks if I'm sure; I say, "Yes," and she—the good Dr. Burtness—never mentions it again.

Hospitalized Again

~ It's Halloween, and two embarrassed nurses are standing beside my bed. There's something they want to ask, but they don't seem able to do it. Finally, Charlotte spits it out. "Is that," she says, pointing with her pen to a spot somewhere over my head, "natural hair loss? Or is that chemo?" I assure her that it's the handsome kind of hair loss, purely natural, highly sought-after, the kind to which she—and most less fortunate creatures—can only aspire.

In fact, I'm about to tell her how my father's family was worried that too many of my mom's brothers had retained their cranial fuzz and there was a possibility that our beautiful baldness might be compromised in the next generation, but good fortune prevailed, and, oh, by the way, where was my pate wax?

But enough about me.

• • •

I'm back in the hospital. Fevers, pain, vanishing white blood cells, and bingo! Here I am. The fever is the baking-bread kind; you can feel the moisture leaving your dough and the crust forming. They're trying to figure out the bug responsible so that they can match the antibiotic to the biote. All in all, not good news. I attend my daily session of radiation. It's number thirty—five to go.

It turns out that chemo depresses your white blood cell production, and since white blood cells are the main vehicle for fighting infection, your chances of picking up an infection are increased. The signs of an infection are also curbed by your therapies, so fever is really the only signal that something's wrong. Be grateful they caught it, they say.

All right, I'll be grateful.

The worst news is that of all the possible nurse costumes that might have entertained me this Halloween, the ones I'm looking at are pajamas with little panda prints.

J is tired of nagging me to eat and drink. She suggests that we make use of my chest-mounted port to introduce some water. Infuse yourself, she suggests. Bypass the rebellious throat and pour that water right down the vein. Later, she tells me that this home infusion probably saved my life, it's covered by insurance, and a nice nurse comes daily until you learn how to do it yourself and then weekly with supplies.

SHIT! They Canceled My Radiation

No radiation today. In order to help my poor, sagging body get its white blood cell count back up, they canceled today's radiation. They may even shave a bit of the dose off the last chemo packet. Why would I be upset about missing out on a zap? Well, they just tack another day on at the end.

Pulmonary Embolism?

It's not a school of medieval theology, although I like imagining the Pulmonary Embolists arguing fiercely with the Chronic Rheumatists. I imagine them fulminating, creaking, and finally burning each other at the stake.

Too bad: pulmonary embolism is a big, fat blood blockage that grows in your lung. People with cancer who sit on their malignant butts often develop clots in the legs that migrate to the lungs. That's what they're worried about, and that's what lands me on the disabled list for the radiotherapy team. If it turns out that I have clots in lungs or legs, we have a whole new set of problems.

Hospitalized

Hospitalized: it's one hell of a word. We understand it as referring to "beginning a stay in a hospital," but it just as easily carries the seeds of "turning into a hospital-compatible creature" and is on a par with "winterized" and "customized." And, sure enough, a few days in a room with motorized beds and you start to fit in to the landscape.

After four days here, I'm getting used to carrying around the pole that supports my IV; I offer my arm up meekly for the cuff or puncture of the moment. I already have a port that gives them instant access to a vein, and it seems like all I need now is the feeding tube and custom-made wheelchair. I can't eat or drink and all they ask is what I want for dinner.

I get released on the fifth day, all hydrated and shiny, and fortunately not thoroughly hospitalized.

• • •

They're letting me go because there are no clots to deal with. The docs decide that it's just a case of pneumonia, so they've prescribed an antibiotic. The game has definitely been postponed, however, and now we'll get to learn the rules about starting up again.

Radiation Day Number Thirty-Five

∼ There's a bell mounted on a wooden plaque in the radiation treatment area. The attached inscription suggests that you should ring the bell when your treatment's done. The bell is the common and essential musical instrument in Tibetan Buddhist rituals, and if you ever want to make a JuBu (Jewish Buddhist) feel right at home, just bring out the bell and give her a ring. The hollow of the bell symbolizes the fact that wisdom is not separated from emptiness.

In Buddhist rituals, the bell is tied to the dorje, or clapper. The bell represents wisdom, the female principle, and the dorje represents compassion or activity, the masculine principle. The sound of the bell is taken to be the speech of the Buddha.

You can imagine my attraction to this bell hanging here in Radiation Alley, even allowing for the fact that this plaque was probably designed to thank "Buck" Bulkholster for his twenty-two years of service to Lodge Number Six and intended to be sold in the Trophy-While-U-Wait section of your local discount store.

Yup, I've been thinking about that bell a lot. This is the place where my spiritual and active selves could get together—the place where cancer could collapse and vanish. Yowsa, man, there's a new life in the sound.

So, I grab the bell, somehow already hearing the one perfect note. I feel the tension in my pecs and deltoids, a wiggle in my forearm, a squeeze of fingers on rope, and a perfect cancer note as I slam the male, active principle into the receptive shell.

When I strike it, the goddamn bell breaks. Pieces go flying all over, wall to wall. (It's the clapper that breaks, you know. It's always the clapper's fault. I'm told that in Tibet there are women who make a nice living describing various sorts of humorous dorje-clapper failure.)

The bell rings, of course, and the sound is perfect, and there are some great little clanks and dinks as the small crowd scurries around picking up pieces of fugitive bings and fragments of runaway bongs. (I like the image of a runaway bong . . .) And everybody shakes my hand, and nobody hands me a bill for a bell, and, yes, I can still hear it ringing.

Ten Days Later

The end of radiation and chemotherapy seems like a milestone. No more daily trips, no more reflections of your diminishing self on politely polished surfaces. Unfortunately, it's not much of a turning point in the way you feel. No, in the shimmering "now" in which this all takes place, ten days after radiation has you feeling a little bit worse. You're weaker and stupider, too. Information makes its way into your center reluctantly, as if it knew it was going to be dealt with badly. Conversations aren't finished, connections aren't made, and ideas—if you have them at all—just sort of flop around and die like bugs that emerge too soon in spring.

But this ain't spring. It's mid-November in Mt. Airy, cold and dim. My only encouragements come from my friends, my agent, and my guardian angel. J. R. has briskly decided that a manuscript of mine is worth her talents and needs just a nip and a tuck in the style department. I don't quite have the wit to do the work, but I'm enjoying her assigned reading, and I think that I'm revived enough now to know what style means.

So, maybe this is the bottom. Maybe today's the worst; stay tuned.

Returning Diminished

Until my diagnosis, I was a minor-league gym rat. Not a serious bodybuilder, mind you, but a ten-to-twelve-times-a-month Pump Addict. Here's how it went: after a half hour or so of biking or rowing, I'd find my weights and my bench. I'd remember a posture, and in a few seconds, I'd close out the world. My attention, no, my whole consciousness sat in a loose wrap around the muscles that were about to work. Then I'd let my breath out as I started the first movement. My mind would tighten around the muscle; everything else would fade away.

I'd let the weight go back to the beginning. That's one repetition (a rep, in the lingo). Without pausing, I'd start the second rep and let my mind melt into the muscle. By the sixth or eighth or tenth rep, I'd be lost in the exhaustion of the muscle, half-dissolving into the feeling of total depletion. That's one set of reps.

Most exercises got three to five sets, with a pause between sets to allow the muscle to recover. At the end of the last rep of the last set, there would be no me and no muscle, just the place where we met and the explosion of the effort. When I stopped, what I could feel was the ump, a surging, singing rush into the muscles. After six or seven different exercises, my whole body would be ringing: pumped.

My last real workout was in mid-September; let's call it nine weeks ago. I stopped because I felt weak and tired, and it was just easier to stop. Today I went back for the second time. I did about twelve minutes on a stationary bike and then went to the bench press. That's an exercise where you lie flat and use the big muscles of the chest and arms to push up a weight and lower it slowly. I reduced the amount of weight that I used to use by half, I began the movement, and all I could feel was something outside of the muscle straining to lift, struggling with the very idea of push. I stopped and reduced the weight by half again. Less strain this time, but the same artificial feeling of watching some guy push weight around. Needless to say, no pump.

I'm figuring that it's a practice effect—that there's something that my body forgot and that it needs to be reminded gently and with good humor. I'll be going back tomorrow—stay tuned.

Grateful: Thanksgiving

Back when I was married, we used to have a Thanksgiving ritual. Before we ate, we'd go around the table and each person would say what he or she was grateful for.

So, here goes:

I'm grateful to J, who has met a lot of challenges these last two months. I'm grateful to all the friends who help me get to treatments. I'm grateful to all the friends who keep in touch—their kindness makes me want to cry sometimes. I'm grateful that my kid is relatively unscarred by all this.

I'm grateful for my dog. I'm grateful that I avoided the feeding tube. I'm grateful that you don't have cancer.

The Way to Save

You gotta hand it to cancer: it's a real money-saver, a veritable fountain of thrift. Check this out. It's been about ninety days since I started treatment, and look at the money I've saved:

With some help, I used to go through four or five bottles of wine a week. At Pennsylvania prices, that's about $1,000 in the course of ninety days.

There's not much dining out when you can't chew, so, conservatively, that's another $600 in the bank. We haven't done much damage to the fancy beer lately, either, let's say $180 there.

Whatever shopping impulses I might have had have gone dormant, so that's $100 or so, and I haven't spent anything on clothes, which saves at least another $10. Oh, and of course there's the matter of razor blades. There's no shaving when the X-rays cut your whiskers off, so that's another $8, maybe $9.

So, put it all together and that's $1,898 still in my bank account that otherwise would have ended up supporting Philadelphia's hospitality industry.

Pretty miraculous, huh? If you ask me nicely, I may also explain about the miracle cancer diet. It really melts the fat right off of you. Really.

· · ·

From a Letter I Wrote to an Austrian Friend in Cambridge Who's Finishing up Grading Papers:

I am still mostly self-absorbed in my struggle to recover from the medical treatments. It's all profoundly boring and blatantly unavoidable. What's up right now is that I can't taste or even eat in a normal way. The radiation is beamed right at the salivary glands, which dry up and stop producing. Aside from a chronically dry mouth being pretty annoying—it can wake you up in the middle of the night—it means that chewing doesn't prepare food to be digested; it just crumbles it up. The dry, crumbly food isn't swallowable—you need moisture. In the end it seems that all eating is really drinking. The condition is called xerostomia.

The same dryness seems to destroy taste—I guess the taste buds work best when wet—so there is little pleasure in the eating I do. Instead, meals have become a sort of game. I total up the calories consumed and try to get to a number that will help me regain some of the weight and muscle that I lost.

When I look in the mirror, I see a loose-fleshed, plucked bird. Thanksgiving just having passed, the image is not a fortunate one. Friends tell me how good I look, but that's what friends do, I suppose. Sleeves that once stretched to accommodate my arms now hang loosely—I think they look a little sad, but maybe I'm projecting.

My diet is built around a dairy-based commercial drink called Ensure. The vanilla version is the least offensive. I eat some mandarin oranges, which come with their own liquid, and I make mousse au chocolate, which dissolves very nicely on the tongue. There are a few other drinks and some concoctions out of the blender that enable me to liquefy what should be solid and fool my throat into accepting it. I also borrowed a juicer, and I buy big bags of carrots and celery in the Italian market. I have become a de facto vegetarian—the thought of blending up a chicken thigh or a lamb loin makes me want to gag—and I guess I should be grateful for the attendant karma.

My Internet sources say that the changes are probably permanent—one doesn't recover from xero-whatever that's induced by radiation. My doctors are more optimistic; they say that something—spit or sensibility—may return. They talk about three months or so. I'll keep you posted.

Radiation Day Number Thirty-Five

I'm not writing a thing. Not a single poem, although I do have a book of poetry being published next month by Thunderclap Press. (It's called *BOOM!* subtitled *Poems for a Certain Generation*.) I have some food writing that I could get to, but the thought of writing about food now seems like bullshit: a man living on industrial human feed shouldn't (or maybe can't) wax persuasive about the joys of learning to cook for oneself.

I'd love to know about the results of your wine tasting. I'm always glad to hear that the wine fields are expanding, for that means that wine has a chance to become more of a daily delight and less of a precious treat. I can't imagine, though, how Austria could be outdone by "other countries"; I'm still a fierce partisan of Burgenland. My interest in wine has become mostly academic— my poor, arid mouth can barely stand to have a sip of wine in it. I don't know if it's the acid or the tannins, but what I experience is an unpleasant burn. I can enjoy a single glass of beer, though, and when I do, I can pick out some of the old, familiar flavors. If I brew again, I'll make something low in carbonation to be easier on the tongue.

Me, Mike Douglas, and a Certain Cancer

～ Nothing metastasizes in a vacuum: the news story that's playing like a soundtrack for my little adventure is the accounting of the cancer of Michael Douglas, the actor. Like me, he has head and neck cancer—stage four—and, according to the stories, he—like me—has an 80 percent chance of living through it.

His story and mine have some other parallels—we're the same age, we're the same ethnicity, we both have beautiful life partners, and we both seem to have enjoyed a pretty good time so far. Sure, I missed out on the fame, fortune, and Hollywood part, and (poor Mike) he probably never crossed the ocean in a sailboat, taught culinary school in Italy, or saw the Dodgers play at Ebbets Field. Six o' one, I say—no reason for him to feel jealous. We're both getting great care, and neither of us is entitled to rail against cruel fate.

There's one other thing we have in common: both of us trooped in and out of doctors' offices with a set of symptoms for a long time before anybody said, "Hey, that's cancer!" I'll bet Mike had the earaches and the sore throats. Maybe he even found himself spitting up bits of blood from time to time. Chances are that someone snaked a tube down his nose, too, and looked around and didn't see the cancer that was growing there. Didn't see it until it became a dome light flashing "stage four," blocking traffic in the middle of his life.

Me, Mike Douglas, and a Certain Cancer

So, here are some things that are puzzling about this whole business, some questions that I'm thinking Mike and I might both want to get answered:

- What makes this cancer so hard to see? Is there anything Mike or I could have done? Is there some chance that the doctors who looked at my sore throat and missed this diagnosis could give some thought to what went wrong? What can we all do now to help make this mistake less likely for other people?
- That 80 percent survival rate is important. It that suggests that both of us have cancers that started with an HPV infection—a sexually transmitted condition. (Regular squamous cell cancer of the head and neck has a lower survival rate.)

HPV by itself doesn't necessarily lead to cancer. In most people it's harmless. The body fights off the infection, and the virus becomes inactive. Certain HPV strains lead to warts, annoying but not malignant. Other HPV strains are deemed "high-risk" because they occasionally develop into a persistent infection that can progress to cervical cancer in women and head and neck cancer in men.

It turns out that HPV is one of the few cancers that can be prevented with a vaccine. Right, a vaccine. Like the ones for mumps and chicken pox. Should we (Mike and I) make a big deal out of this? Should we use our star power to tell the world that there's a cancer that's preventable with a vaccine? That we got it, but you don't have to? Should we mention that these HPV cancers could be stamped out in a generation?

Maybe Mike and I should take this little moment to suggest[§] that anyone with children ask their doctor about Cervarix and

---

§ In the interest of full disclosure: Although the opinions expressed and faulty thinking promulgated here are entirely the author's, Our Lady of the Sick Coincidence has fixed it so that J, my mainstay, was employed for a time by the manufacturer of the most effective HPV vaccine.

Gardasil, the two vaccines that are proven to prevent HPV when they're given before a person becomes sexually active. We could do a commercial together (although I might have to coach him on how to say his lines).

- One other thing: if we each have an 80 percent chance of making it, there's a 64 percent chance that we'll both make it. When we do, Mike, I'll buy you a drink.

Chocolate Mousse for the Recently Radioactive

Swallow This:

Eating is really drinking, so if you don't make enough liquefy-
ing saliva of your own, you'd better figure out how to put things
in your mouth that are already wet. That gives you a menu of
blender drinks and supplements and, after a few weeks, a diet
of boredom. But there is one thing that goes in your mouth dry
and light and then dissolves into creamy liquid goodness all by
its own chemistry—it's mousse au chocolate (or chocolate pudding, if you hate the French).

I've been making it, and I don't see any reason why you shouldn't,
too. Why should the sick guy have all the fun?

Here's what you do: separate two eggs, putting the whites in a
large bowl and the yolks in a cup. Make sure that you don't get even
a speck of yolk in with the whites. Measure out two or three ounces
of chocolate (figure on using a candy bar's worth), and put it in a
small dish and then in the microwave. Melt the chocolate in short
bursts, stirring each time. You don't want the chocolate to get too
hot, or it will cook the eggs when you add them.

When the chocolate is melted, whip the egg whites until they
form stiff peaks—a minute or so with a handheld electric mixer.
Be sure not to whip them back into a liquid. Add a tablespoon of
Myers's rum and half a tablespoon of really good vanilla extract to

the egg whites. If your doctor is one of those humorless medics who forbids alcohol, add an ounce of very, very strong coffee—don't be afraid to use a bit of instant coffee to intensify the flavor. The stiff foam of the whites will collapse, but don't worry about it.

Add the egg yolks to the melted chocolate and stir them in. Then pour the chocolate–egg yolk mixture into the egg whites and gently stir them together until you have a light brown mix. Pour this stuff (we can call it mousse now) into cups and refrigerate for an hour or so until they set. You can multiply this recipe: as long as you keep a half an ounce to an ounce of chocolate per egg, you'll be fine.

If you picked a good chocolate, what you have is magic. Dry turns to moist, and chocolate explodes in your mouth. Of course, the better the chocolate, the better the mousse, so don't be stingy. Even if nothing else has tasted good in a while, you may actually enjoy your food for a minute or two—a good thing whether you have cancer or not.

The Verdict

It's easy to forget that all this life-squelching radiation and platinum infusions have a purpose. They're supposed to kill the tumor before it kills me. It's easy to forget about the tumor because the cure is itself a disease, and the recovery from that disease is right here in my life and every day.

But we're about to find out if all this was to any purpose. On Thursday, I go for a CAT scan of the tumor, which was living and growing just under my right jaw. There are three possible outcomes, three potential headlines to be generated by the scan. One is that it was all for nothing, and it's time to kiss my ass goodbye. Two is that the thing is dead, and I'm going to live. The third is that there's still too much inflammation from the X-rays to be able to tell, and we have to wait another eight weeks and look again.

My daughter asks me if I'm nervous about the outcome, and I tell her that I'm not. For one thing, I can feel that the tumor has shrunk and that its influence has diminished. More importantly, there's nothing to be nervous about. The job is done, the votes have been cast, and there's nothing to do but read the results. In the meantime, there's just now and questions about what kind of chocolate to put in the truffles that I'm bringing to somebody's party this weekend. Back when I got the diagnosis—stage four, you may remember—I pretty much wrote off the rest of life, so if there's news, it will be good, and if the outcome is bad, well, that's not news.

As I said to Archibald McLeish and Tina Turner just the other day, "Don't Cry for Me, Arch and Tina." And that's what I say to you, too.

• • •

Here's a curious side bit on The Verdict. The doctors told me that they'd do the scan on Thursday and tell me the results the following Tuesday. I wondered, whispering the question—what the point of the five-day delay was.

"Does it take that long to read the CAT scan?"

"No, it's just that we don't have clinic again until Tuesday."

"Are you telling me that someone will know my fate on Thursday, and I won't know until a week later?" (Notice how I used my indignation to inflate five days into a week.)

Doctors are really cute when they're caught looking guilty, so—after some staring at the floor and shuffling of the feet—one of them thought it over and allowed that I could call on Friday and he'd tell me the results. Good man.

• • •

Occasionally someone I haven't seen in a while asks, "What going on?" or "How the heck are you?" and I have to give a serious answer. On days when I have a voice at all , there's a certain tone to my answer. The note is a touch defensive, as if the questioner had a right to be disappointed. What? You? Cancer? Oh. Maybe it's shame or at least embarrassment.

That's the problem with all this rah-rah stuff about having the right attitude in the face of The Monster. If the right attitude will kill the tumor, what the hell was wrong with your attitude that you got it in the first place?

Actually, someone has looked into this. At the University of Pennsylvania, they followed a thousand patients with "good attitude" and another thousand with "bad attitude." It turns out there wasn't much difference in survival rates. Of course "survival" is the wrong measure here. What's really going on is that people with good attitude live with a good attitude: a nice way to live, even with cancer.

Tricks

The CAT scan for the tumor is over in a matter of minutes. May I see the images? No, you may not, we have more patients to deal with. Very well, then.

On the way back to my car, I feel the lump in my jaw. Is it bigger? Maybe. Then I notice that my throat is sore—right in the spot where the tumor was discovered. And then there's that earache, just like the one that I had before treatment.

Time to think about something else.

It's Inconclusive

I got a call from Dr. Skarbnik, the junior of my two oncologists. Here's what he found out: the lymph node under my jaw is cleared of cancer, but there is still a two-centimeter malignant mass on my tongue.

My next appointment is with the surgeon, and we all know what surgeons think is the best solution. The surgery could leave me unable to speak, and it will certainly ruin the headshots I use when I audition for major motion picture roles. Dr. Skarbnik holds out the possibility that another round of chemotherapy may do the trick.

I have no way of knowing what the probabilities are—the chemo option may be just a way of softening the blow.

In the meantime, I'm going to use the small voice I have left to say, "I love you," and "Good dog!" and "You really did a good job." What will you use yours for?

The End of Optimism

Every time I got strapped down to the radiation rig, I thought that I was going to be lucky: that the X-rays and the chemicals would work and I would be clear of cancer when they were done. I fantasized about going on with my life with this episode fading slowly into the background until it became an anecdote. I imagined the whole thing being diluted by other concerns until my memory of the stories of treatment became more real than my memories of the treatment itself. I almost envisioned telling my grandchildren. It was a quiet, robust optimism—the power of positive radiation made plain, and it was dead wrong.

The vision now is that either I'm really messed up by the surgery and that I will then carry on in that condition until I'm either cured or killed by the tumor, or I simply skip the surgery and let the thing progress. The advantage of the latter course is that I have more time in a relatively healthy—or at least intact—condition. The Fox Chase website warns that the surgery interferes with eating, breathing, and talking, three activities that I've grown to love. There's also a wonderful sentence on the site about trying to avoid "breaking the jaw or splitting the lip" during surgery, and I fervently wish them good luck with that. I'll have to find out how radical the surgery will be before I choose.

In eight days, I see the surgeon. Lots of time to think about things, like what to do, bucket lists, life summaries, who gets the cookbooks, stuff like that. I'll keep you posted.

Whiplash, or Everything You Know Is Wrong

J is unhappy. It seems to her that someone should know more than they're letting on about my diagnosis and that I shouldn't have to wait two weeks to find out what's next.

So she calls the oncologist for a little doctor-to-doctor chat. (I called this person last week. All I got was a nurse returning my call, saying, "Shut up and show up.") Anyway, when the grown-ups put their heads together, there's a slightly different version of reality.

First, it turns out that more chemo isn't an option. "Studies show" that the amount I got was the right amount and anything additional is just toxic to the patient.

The mass that remains on my tongue might be malignant, or it might be just scar tissue and inflammation. The purpose of the visit to the surgeon is to find out what that little two centimeters is all about. He's going to stick his fist down my throat, maybe attach a periscope, perhaps strap on a scuba tank, and go in for the biopsy. I'm not too sanguine: the thing was quiet all during treatment and for four weeks afterward. Scar tissue wouldn't start growing after lying dormant for a while, would it?

What are the probabilities one way or the other? Again, any reference to "chance" or "probability" makes the line go dead silent. J doesn't know; she says that because my tumor was HPV-dependent, the science is all new. I think she's covering for her profession, but I'm glad that she could make the call and grateful that she did. Me? I'm still balanced on a knife edge, just a slightly different one.

The funny thing (ha ha) is that I'm not rooting for an outcome, not fantasizing getting a pass and skipping out of the surgeon's office singing. I'm just waiting, walking the dog, writing to you, editing a novel that I hope will see the light of ink, and thinking about a bucket list.

• • •

I woke up around noon, walked to the bathroom, and passed out on the way. When I came to, I called Hugh Gilmore. I got downstairs; maybe I wobbled, maybe I flew. Dunno. Something about unlocking the door so whoever it is doesn't have to break it down. Breaking down is bad.

Gilmore drove me to Fox Chase. When J arrived, I asked her if this was the part where I die. She said, "No," but the transition from conscious to un- was so easy, so cancerish that it seemed like a perfectly reasonable question at the time.

More on my bucket list tomorrow.

The Incredible
Shrinking Lynn

~⌐ My friend Hugh Gilmore wrote this in his column, *Enemies of Reading*. It's about watching me shrink:

> And each day, this muscular guy who started out with a big torso and thick arms slipped farther into his shirt and jacket, until by the culminating 35th day of radiation he looked like a little kid wearing his big brother's clothes.

(I'm surprised at my little rush of vanity as I read this. Me? Muscular? Golly.)

And my dear friend Brenda—the mother of my godchildren— writes from deepest Mississippi that she's reluctant to call for fear of disturbing me. When the bell on the phone is too much for you, you've really shrunk.

Here's what I think about life while you're waiting:

clothes call

through the hospital halls, jaws locked, eyes straight ahead
march the lock-legged legions of the sick in clothes they wore
when they were well. costumed each as a former self.
All wrapped up in yesterday sinking through today
with collar buttons on chests and pleated waists
and sleeves rolled up to where their hands end.

On the street outside, the man with two kids shows off

RADIATION DAYS

his teenage jacket, boyhood pants.
the lady who left her husband last year does her hair
like it was on her wedding day.
the off-duty cop flashes the chains as he sports
for stuff and something on the street.
the priest goes by in his jogging suit
point guard for the gospel according to.
the bhikku wraps his saffron robe
in winter tweed and suffers not a whit.

And then the bell strikes one, two, three
and everyone strips off their past
and stares blinking in the fierce light of now
and someone—the cop? the lady?
starts to giggle and the bhikku smiles
and then the hospital echoes like a horn filled up
with its own music as Extra Large hits the floor
and Medium, naked, begins to laugh.

Mardical Medijuana—An Op-Ed Submission

〜 I'm in my sixties, which means I was in my twenties in the seventies, which were really the sixties—if you catch my drift. One of the legacies of that Golden Age is a healthy skepticism about drugs.

Skepticism? Don't you mean belief? Reverence?

Well, no. The first thing that we learned about drugs was that Mom, Dad, our high school basketball coach, our teacher, our preacher, and our dear over-reacher all friggin' lied to us about pot. They said it was bad; we knew it was good, and even though they threw millions of dollars of research money away, they were never able to pin much of anything on it. A harmless pleasure.

As you know, a victimized harmless pleasure can easily be turned into a rite of defiance. (What do you suppose motivates the Iranian women who carelessly show a bit of well-cared-for *hair*?)

So we made marijuana into a miracle and smoked it into a virtue, and the company of the virtuous became our family, and that's the subject for a poem or two, maybe even a chapbook of 'em.

And now I have cancer—head and neck. It's stage four, spreading out across the base of my tongue, and what matters most from this end of the biopsy is that Mary Jane has a reputation as a cancer fighter. She suppresses nausea, increases appetite, and otherwise puts a pleasant, companionable smile on things. Just a few days ago, I was nauseated, weak, and miserable at the thought of having a feeding tube inserted into my chest. I was sick and teetering on the edge of depression. Even if I hadn't remembered that pot was a weapon against all this, my friends would have reminded me. In just about every "I got cancer" conversation, the question came up: "You going to try medical marijuana?"

In my initial meeting with Dr. Burtness, the oncologist, I asked about medical marijuana. Dr. B. allowed that some people get some relief from a drug called Marinol, but she was skeptical. (Marinol is pot with all the fun taken out.)

I should jump back here to tell you that this was the lady who, in taking my medical history, asked me if I "used" alcohol. I replied that I "used" shaving cream, frying pans, and a power sander, but that I delighted in a long relationship with alcohol that had left us both the better for it.

Yes, it sounded almost as pompous as it reads, but the delivery was softened by my Brooklyn accent and therefore slightly more lovable than garrulous. To her credit, she laughed.

Dr. Burtness's skepticism and mine in perfect pole-for-pole symmetry resulted in my standing in the kitchen a few days ago poaching a wad of decent homegrown pot in butter. The THC in the pot is soluble in fat, see, so when I use the butter to make, um, let's say, some vanilla shortbread, what I get is a cookie that has designs on you, a bonbon to bite you back.

I ate my first one just after my noontime visit to radio land. In a half hour there was this little premonitory rumble. In an hour, I had exceeded Mach 1 while sitting on the edge of my bed. The first thing I have to tell you is that appetite and nausea are not problems anymore. The Munchies are alive and well; although they are a bit disappointed that we've been neglecting them, they're glad to see us, and they're willing to talk about it.

Yes, for the first time in six weeks or so, I felt hungry. Fruit, yogurt, hummus, salad, juice, ice cream. The metal taste was gone, and things tasted pretty much like themselves. Wine? A swallow of Fatty Boombalatty was a bit too tart going down, but a sip of Zaccagnini's Riserva Monte was like music and laughter at the same time. Nausea? Who's she?

As for the pleasant, companionable smile, I think it's time to take the dog to the woods. As soon as I finish dancing around the room to Dr. John.

So, now, it's tomorrow, although it's today—of course you knew that. I had a little nibble of pot-spiked shortbread before I went to my radiation treatment. Bzzz. Smooth as silk. Home now with a big lunch under my belt, I'm sleepy, happy, and puzzled. I'm happy to be sleepy, happy to feel like a living being again, happy to have some energy, and thrilled that I'm having fantasies about what kind of kayaking I want to do when this is all over.

What I'm puzzled about is this: who the hell objects so strenuously to sick people feeling better?

Ooo, ooo, wait, I know! Mom, Dad, our high school basketball coach, our teacher, our preacher, and so on. They lied back then, and they're lying to us now. Marijuana helps sick people feel better, ain't that so, brothers and sisters? Say, "Amen."

• • •

Pamela is one of my dog-walking friends, she of the silky black dog named Mica. She leaves a big pot of soft, creamy-bland, comforting

RADIATION DAYS

soup in a tureen by the front door. One of a dozen kindnesses that
climb up out of the neighborhood to find me.

The Bucket List

～ When I started thinking about a bucket list, I surprised myself. There wasn't much on it, and what was there was none too dramatic. This may be a sign of a life well-led or just a lack of imagination—I'll leave that call to you. But I don't really get skydiving, I'd like to travel but don't feel a lust for any place in particular, and—aside from Terry Gross and "Marty" Moss-Coane—I've already met everyone I want to know, thank you.

This may be the foundation of a critique of the BL idea itself. Why wait for a bad diagnosis to do what you want? What's stopping you now, pilgrim?

The one thing that comes to mind—one itch that I've had for a while—is that I'd like to get rid of my stuff and die owning a pocket knife, a cast iron skillet, and an iPhone. More or less.

Part of this impulse stems from my own weird animism: I worry for my poor little books and antiques and art supplies. Who will take care of them? Will they feel sad? (Yes, it's not for nothing that this is called the Pathetic Fallacy.)

Another part is that I imagine my daughter facing a house full of crap and not having much time to deal with it. I imagine the dumpster outside the door filled with daguerreotype cameras, pastel sticks, and rubber-stamp-type kits. It all seems like such a waste.

RADIATION DAYS

I played with this idea in a poem—published this year in *Urban Legends*—that has this bit at the beginning:

> I dream that my house catches fire.
> Not a little fire—that would be a pain in the ass.
> I mean a real level—the motherfucker inferno,
> a light-up-the-sky, smell it in Camden
> con-fla-smokin'-gration.

And also contains this:

> Now the fantasy heats up (so to speak).
> All of the crap I've brought back to my nest
> One flight at a time
> is suddenly transformed into pure choice.
> No thing left, just possibilities.
> Vaporized nouns leave me solid verbs behind.

There's more to my bucket list, but that's enough for today. It's made me a little sad: sort of like having to leave the party early or losing touch with a friend. It's stopped snowing, and I think I'll walk the dog again.

Life Summary— Preliminary Considerations

∾ As I think about writing a life summary, there's a crew cutting down the Norway maples across the street in Fairmount Park. This is a good thing because these invasive trees very quickly crowd out the native species and in the process choke off the food supply on which our native bugs and birds and mammals depend. Left to itself, our forest would be replaced in fifty years or so by a sterile tree plantation.

The tree service contractors won't get them all—even I can see three big ones that they missed. These survivors will drop seed and outgrow and sun-starve the natives around them, and in a few years all the good work will be undone.

It would be sweet to think about permanent solutions to the problem of the dying forest, and here's the way I think about it now:

norway maple in fairmount park

it's mostly the muscles that want to swing
the axe that whacks at the base of the forest-killing weed tree.
as much as you think you know about the death of the
woods and the invading foreigners starving out
the birds and bugs and butterflies,
it's really the sound
as it echoes off your bark
and the hard deceleration of the axe as you feel it leaf

RADIATION DAYS

through the wood of your arms and into your trunk
and the tickle of the trickle of sweat along your ribs
as you make the first warm day of spring.

the day after you salted the stumps and planted
the little oaks and beeches and wild blueberry,
they sent a crew out into the neighborwoods and asked each household:
"Did you hear those norway maples fall?
Did you see the sun again on the forest floor?"
And when it turned out that no one did, you went back
to the woods and there—the norway maples unchopped and arrogant,
not caring about your axe or the pathetic fallacy,
sneering at the doomed little oaks,
knowing quite well that no one was listening
and they, therefore, were quite safe.

later, later when the woods had died
and the last fox tripped starving through
the plantation that we let in place where
the woods would wood,
you had to wonder:
is swinging the axe
and a tired back all that ever mattered?
are the sweat and the sound the only
wages of the day?
and if they are—
where do you go and
who do you thank for that?

(This poem got published two years later in *Everyday Poets*.)

Part of me roots for the forest; another part is happy just that they're doing the work. So how shall I make my own life summary? Is it a list of forests saved or a list of days spent happily chopping?

Tomorrow at Fox Chase

~ Tomorrow I see the surgeon. Aboard the SS *Cancer*, the surgeon is the captain of the ship, the one who steers the course, the one who helps you avoid overdoing the nautical metaphors. In this case, he is the very tall and very imperious Dr. Drew Ridge.

He's the one who's going to tell me where I land on the continuum between cancer-free and hospice-bound. In the middle, there are lots of variations on doing surgery: some of the surgical possibilities are high-tech and relatively bloodless; some of them look like something you'd do to a farmyard animal.

Am I nervous? I don't think so, but I notice that I haven't slept real well for the last few days.

Tonight, to mark the occasion, J and I went out to dinner. We had a seven-fishes tasting menu at one of our favorite restaurants—a joint called Matyson. The seven-fishes is a Roman Christmas tradition. Its backstory involves noble Roman families competing to provide lavish entertainment to the Pope and his entourage. In this country, it's become the property of folks from the South (of Italy). Since it's almost impossible to pull off at home (Seven fish courses in one meal? Get real.) it's a treat to find it in a restaurant.

The highlight was this gorgeous piece of crisp-skinned red snapper on a bed of sweet potato cubes with a few mussels and a broth made from the mussel jus.

J drank Vouvray; I had a bottle of Allagash Tripel (batch 148) that I've been saving for a year or so, waiting for the night before Cancermas to pull the cork. Delicious, spicy, round, and still assertive. It stings my radiation-roughed-up mouth a little, but you could forgive anything for that taste.

And so we toasted. "To you," she said. In a fit of originality, I replied, "No, to you." And then we both agreed on "To tomorrow."

Bad News/Good News

Bad news gets to you slowly in Cancerland, kind of like a Caribbean squall that you see coming toward you in the distance as you tack upwind. Dr. Ridge looks, feels, tries to get past my gag reflex to feel around, and quits. He says that it could be scar tissue, could be tumor.

I knew that. So, doc, what's the chances of tumor? Can't say. What happens if there is a tumor? Surgery. How bad is the surgery? It's rough; you'll meet with the reconstructive surgeons beforehand to talk about repairs.

Reconstructive surgery? That suggests that there's going to be some destruction first—some vandalism on the side of my head. This was when I had the "blood runs cold" feeling, that sense of ice in the chest.

"Of course, it could be scar tissue."

"Umm, how often does someone have thirty-five days of radiation and then wait five weeks and have scar tissue clogging his throat?"

"Not often."

"So, we're probably looking at surgery, right?"

"We'll know for sure after a biopsy."

It's scheduled for December 30.

The Future

∽ At a time like this, how do you think about the future? How do you make even the simplest plans? So far, I've figured out two rules. One is that you don't make any promises that you can't be reasonably sure of keeping. No lecture commitments next spring, no cruises booked for Valentine's Day.

The second rule is that—in order to avoid complete paralysis—you have to keep two things in mind:

- You're going to live

and

- You're going to die

If you can keep those two thoughts in mind, it shouldn't take long before you realize that they're both true and always were.

The net is this: sometimes you act on thought number one, sometimes on number two. Either way, you can't go wrong, and, best of all, each mode of thinking spices up the other.

So, I ordered the stuff to build another kayak, and I set up my kid to start renting out my house. And I made sure that someone will take care of the dog.

I have this silly idea that, somehow, somebody should get some good out of my dying, that I should be able to figure out a way for it to be a payoff for somebody—and that there's not a lot of time. It's like having a term paper due tomorrow or realizing that the roast is almost done and you haven't a goddamn idea about what to do for a sauce. I figure it's mostly a matter of making it a gift for my kid and my friends so that somehow when they think about dying (and you gotta think about that from time to time), they think of surfing down the wave and they think of me and themselves as no different than the stuff of stars and oceans and that somehow there's an elegance to the thought. But I don't quite have the way to say this yet, and the clock, well, the price of time gets higher with each tick.

Correspondence

Dear Lynn,

Back in the States for a few days after nearly two months in China. The Great Cyberwall they have created there prevented me from reaching your blog. You must definitely be an Enemy of the People (Enemy and People have always to be capitalized in China).

big hug,

Julio

Dear Julio,

You know that I was too young to get Senator McCarthy's attention and that I totally failed to make Nixon's enemies list, so this is very good news indeed. I've always wanted to be an enemy, and to be one with a capital E is beyond imagining...

Ti Abbraccio,

Lynn

Merry Christmas!

I decide that I'm going to be alive today by being outside—for a few minutes anyway—and let myself soak in the weather. Just a hint of snow this morning and I'm almost mute. Not with joy or awe, just throat-closed mute. So Lola and I take our walk in Carpenter's Woods, me stopping to lean on trees, her stopping to pee on them. It's a partnership, you know.

When we leave the woods, we can see the few snowflakes, a brighter white against the blue-gray white of the sky to the east. I'm watching the flakes slide sideways and down, thinking ballerinas or maybe a very low-budget snow globe, but she's thinking dogfood and in we go.

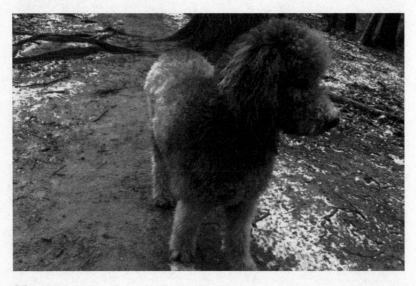

Fling

Tomorrow's the biopsy, and J decided that we should have a little fling in the face of whatever's coming next. So, we went home, to New York, to the place where we were young and always will be. The two things we both love are art and food, so we planned for museums and restaurants and a food court or two.

We spent a whole day at the Met. (That's the Metropolitan Museum of Art for you out-of-towners.) This is the view from one of the better tables at the Met's wine bar.

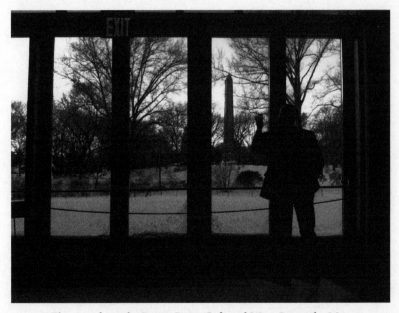

The view from the Petrie Court Cafe and Wine Bar at the Met.

RADIATION DAYS

The obelisk you see outside is a sixty-eight-foot-tall monument that's called Cleopatra's Needle, although it's one thousand years older than the Liz Taylor lookalike. It's been in that spot since 1881, some seven years before my grandfather showed up in the city. The EXIT sign is purely coincidental, and we won't read anything into it.

• • •

It's almost impossible to come back to Philadelphia from New York without feeling a bit humbled. Philly's a great place to live, and we have some really nice urban stuff here, but New York is imperial. It's the head of an empire; all the nations send their treasures there, and then people come from all over the world to admire them. Oh, what a piece of work is Man(hattan).

Emergency Retraining

≈ For something that's called "surgery," today's operation was pretty easy on the patient. Crack of dawn arrival, answer questions, get undressed, and get unconscious. (The anesthesiologist turned out to be a fellow brewer, so there was some shop talk in there.) An hour and change later, you wake up groggy with a wicked sore throat and a keen desire for breakfast and a nap. Your escort takes you home and puts you to bed. If you're lucky, she's beautiful and she kisses your forehead.

The term of choice for something like this at Fox Chase is "procedure," as if to emphasize its kinship with other procedures like chopping an onion or planing the bevel on a sheer clamp. There's even a suite of rooms called the Short Procedure Unit, although no cutting boards or block planes are on display around the place.

The procedure is called a direct laryngoscopy, or DL, as we old cancer hands say. The sore throat comes from the breathing tube and all the pocket tools that are forced down your throat while you're out. The grogginess is partly the drugs and partly the sleep deprivation that comes from waking up at 5:00 a.m. after a less-than-restful night.

Here's what the procedure netted: nothing. Well, not exactly nothing, but nothing definitive. There was a big, ugly sore down there, but what was it? The good doctor says that it could be an ulcer where the tumor used to be, it could be scar tissue, and it could be the surviving remains of the tumor.

So he snipped out a piece and sent it off to the lab to be frozen and analyzed. I guess that's a procedure, too. The answer to the "could-be" questions above? It will be another week before we know. Stay tuned. I know that I certainly will.

Speaking of answers, I tell Gilmore that I'm looking for the ballerina who knows all about malignancy.

When he looks puzzled, I explain that I want the Cancer Answer Dancer. To his great credit, he doesn't say anything about my deteriorating sense of shame. To mine, I don't add that I'd love to seduce her—you know, be the Cancer Answer Dancer Romancer.

• • •

Cancer or not, you still have to walk the dog. Tonight it wasn't so easy. I usually let go of her leash, tell her to heal,[⁵] and walk to the park. When one of us has had enough, I put out my hand and call, "Touch," and she comes to me. I say, "Give me your face," and she sticks her head in the leash and we go home.

Tonight's problem was that I couldn't say "heel" or much of anything else. It'll probably be a few days until my dog-walking voice returns, and it's still possible that I'll lose it completely sometime soon. So, before we went out, I whistled (no damage to my whistling muscles) and held out a treat, and she came. Two more reps and she had it. Then I stamped my foot and pressed her rear down to a sit and gave her another treat. She got that one on one try: stamp = sit. I held out the collar, she slid her head in, and off we went.

I'd call that procedure an immediate success.

---

⁵Slip of the keyboard there—of course I meant "heel."

Looking Back (or Life Summary—Part Two)

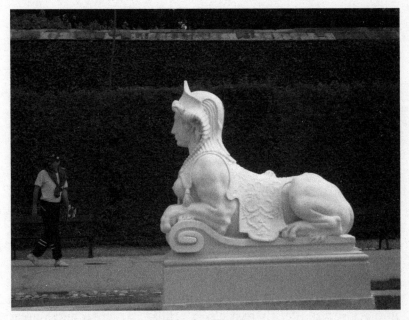

Belvedere-Vienna

∼ There's something pathetic, even tacky about all of the new year–provoked "looking back" features in the press and on the screens. Commentators who are known mostly for their hair being blown around in the wind of the latest fads are suddenly possessed of a sense of history. Sillier yet, things that truly lack a history— like this past NFL season—are suddenly the subject of reflective consideration. What, exactly, are we supposed to learn from "the ten best forward passes of the year"? How about "best celebrity embarrassing moments"?

You get the idea. I'm reluctant to sum anything up for the sake of making a list. I flatter myself when I think that's because I live so much in the present, but maybe my reluctance comes from distress at having to look at the list itself.

At the same time, I find myself drawn to a summary. Maybe it's the clip-clop of the hooves of mortality; maybe it's the pure weasely desire for self-justification.

• • •

So, how did I do with all these years of sucking down oxygen and taking up space? What's my grade? Did I break 700 on the SAT (Substantial Accomplishment Test)?

You may be shocked to hear this: it depends.

A kind way to put it would be that I spent most of my time doing things that I liked and hardly hurt anybody in the process. Along the way, there were five books and twenty years of teaching that were pretty well received. Most of my exes are still talking to me, and a few friends keep in touch. It's a two-column-inch obituary sort of life. There is also a brilliant daughter and a great golden-age romance, but I think myself more lucky than deserving in those instances.

Less kindly, I think that my accomplishments were pretty modest. I lacked the courage or the energy to keep my first marriage together, and my vocational efforts were spread across so many fields as to be diluted to almost homeopathic proportions. I let myself drift away from Art and I was too scared for Drama.

Looking Back (or Life Summary—Part Two)

. . .

So, what it comes down to is this: if I tote up all the nouns in my list of accomplishments, it doesn't look so good. If I consider how I spent my time and the pleasure I gave and satisfaction I took, if I concentrate on the verbs, it's not so bad, after all. (And what should I make of "Great Thanksgiving Dinners Cooked"? The applause on the last day of a class?) How much of an *Apologia* do I need for *Vita Mia*?

It's a heavy question, one that cuts to the heart of what it is to be human. The sun is shining as I write this. I step outside to see, then make some shadows. I have 'til Friday before I meet with the surgeon to get the biopsy results, and J just suggested that we have some sushi. I think I'll go with the verbs.

93

The End of the Road

∼ I should have seen it coming. She was old; she had a leaky valve and more than her share of dings and nicks. I had even fantasized about what life would be like without her. But, still, it's hard to say goodbye to a 1994 Toyota Camry that's served you for 150,000 miles. This was the first car I'd owned after years of Center City living and walking everywhere. It was the one that carried my kid around and the car in which the dog and I drove away from home when it wasn't home anymore.

Of course I know that it's silly to personify a car, but there's an attachment that's bred of reliability and usefulness. Right now, just a day away from getting the news about what's going on in my throat, I feel kind of fragile—I can barely stand the thought of anything else changing.

And yet, change is the law, so it's time to reframe. Maybe I'll come out of this with a clear throat and a new car. Maybe I'll drive down the road singing.

The News

～ You wait for a while in a room with brown speckled plastic wallpaper, recessed lighting, and fake wood floors. There's a rack with machines, an endoscope, some cameras and a monitor, a cabinet below a built-in unit with a sink that looks like it came from a suburban studio apartment. There are two patient chairs, beige things with control units. I find its very banality forbidding—it's a room whose dullness could blunt the sharp keen of somebody wailing.

You wait for the surgeon for a while. There's a range of outcomes here. We could be looking at radical, disfiguring surgery and a feeding tube. There's the heartwarming story on the Fox Chase website of the woman who sewed up a little fanny pack for her husband so that he could carry around the bottle of food that was connected to his feeding tube. Enabled him to play golf, it did. Or we could be over and done, cancer gone, and nothing to do but outlive the results of the radiation and chemotherapy, finish up a novel, build another kayak, and go sailing all summer long.

What we got was something in between. The biopsy was negative, but there is a large sore that may be masking some tumor. In the meantime, the sore is giving me a raw throat and sharp stabbing pains, and they're getting worse. *What's up?* I write the question. I hope my hand on the paper was determined and no-bullshit insistent. Well, they're not sure. Another biopsy would just irritate the throat some more. So we will have another scan in five weeks and another chance to sit in the brown room.

How do I feel? Relieved. Grateful. Numb. Did this really happen?

Pain

～ There is a common code for conveying how much pain an adult patient is having. The health-care worker says, "On a scale of one to ten, with ten being the worst pain you ever felt, how much does it hurt?" I hope you are unfamiliar with it. (There's a different one for kids called the Wong-Baker Scale. It uses a scale of smiley to agonized faces.)

In the few days since we heard that the biopsy was negative, the pain in my ear, throat, and jaw have gotten worse. Right now it's about an eight. The radiation doc and the surgeon were both stumped, and J is puzzled. Infection? No temperature. I'm weak, sleepy all the time. You could say that I'm dreamy, but only if dreams were thick, sloppy retreats from pain.

Oxycontin—God bless it—and Oxycodone—its name be praised— do a pretty good job, but they have their own costs. A virus? Maybe.

My next step is the oncologist, if I can get her on the phone and get someone to speak for me.

Stay tuned; I know I will.

The Job (or Life Summary— Part Three)

～ We've established that even if you have cancer, you continue to walk the dog. It's just as true that your karma continues to walk you.

I got a call a few weeks ago from the dean at the Academy of Culinary Arts. They have a visiting professor slot available—would I like to come visit? Maybe teach courses like Gastronomy and Culture?

I drove down there two days ago—it's in the Pine Barrens on the way to Atlantic City—did a few interviews, lost my voice toward the end, signed some papers and shook some hands, and it's a deal. The drive wore me out, and I'm wondering how I'll be able to keep up my end of the deal. I haven't taught anything more intense than a tasting in a while. I miss it. No, that's not right. I miss myself as a teacher, and I'm very happy to have me back.

One of the best things about this job at this time is that the Dean and her faculty who asked me to come are former students. They took culinary or wine classes with me on the way to getting college degrees. They must have had a good time doing it. In fact, they told me as much and that, my friends, is the best Life Summary I could get right now.

. . .

The Job (or Life Summary—Part Three)

A bonus from all this is that I get to rethink everything I've ever taught. What do I say about food and culture in fifteen hours? What matters? What do I find still exciting after all these years? What would you say about Italian wine if you only had two hours to do it? Or the American lust for meat? The French passion for cheese? How do you talk about the sheer voluptuousness of food when millions of people don't have clean water or sufficient food? How will I talk at all?

Wow. I don't know what I'll say; time to get to work.

A Bright Idea

～ The pain is shimmering up and down the right side of my head. In a couple of weeks it's outrun Oxycontin/Oxycodone's ability to keep it in check. Along with neck, throat, and temporal lobe pain, there's an ache in my right jaw that won't go away. It's sharp, then dull. Like a toothache.

Toothache?

Shit! Could I have a toothache? Could this whole thing be related to a lousy cavity?

This morning I called a neighborhood dentist. She saw me this afternoon. Sure enough, there's a cavity—a big 'un—and, no, it's not big enough or bad enough to be the source of all this pain.

But the good doctor keeps talking, asking questions, taking a moment to think about the answers. Would I mind if she called the oncologist before she dealt with the cavity? Not at all.

At the end of the day, there's a message: would I please call Fox Chase to schedule a punch biopsy? You bet I will.

The Worst Day Yet

~ Saturday's pain is about double Friday's. I can't swallow without wincing, so I can't eat. My hands tremble, I tremble. It's as if my body is scared for me. I can feel my throat closing on the right side, and I'm getting weaker. And my doctors are just telling me to wait.

I'm not scared—I think I'm too drained to feel fear—but I'm sad. Again, it's the sadness of leaving too soon, the party's still going on, spring training in a few weeks, garden catalogs in the mail. (Oh the beauty! Oh the herbs!) It's so cruel to have been getting better and then have it all snatched away. I'm losing three pounds every two weeks.

• • •

My circumstances include not being able to eat a salad. The greens might as well be sawgrass as I work my jaws around a bone-dry mouth and the mixed delicate mini-greens turn into a hard, stringy mortar. My tongue hurts, and eventually my lower jaw gets tired and starts to hurt. The salad greens still don't change at all. It's not swallow material, and while I could amuse myself wondering when the swallows come back, what I really do is pour a glass of milk. I try to use it to down the pounded greens as if they were high-fiber painkillers, and when that doesn't work, I spit them out and have milk for dinner.

101

Life Summary—Part Four

The Would-Be Lepidopterist

You would have known more about butterflies
if you had killed them more and watched them less.
If you had used a killing jar and a scalpel and collected
the various, variegated genitalia
of Nymphs and Satyrs, Blues and Coppers.
You could have been.

But no, you only planted flowers for them to suck
and sheltered the weeds where they laid their eggs
And applauded when you saw them jump into the air
and wink their way along their next performance.
Applauded! (Who the hell were you applauding?)

No eternity for those bugs or you,
Just a messy, scaly, insect stew.
No dry forever on a pin,
Just vanished scale on a dusty wing.

So you don't know much about butterflies,
You even forget their names from time to time.
You can't tell a Painted Lady from an American,
Vanessa cardui from Vanessa whaz-er-name.

All you have left is that stupid, sharp indrawn breath

Life Summary—Part Four

as you see the Mourning Cloak
(arrogant first-bastard of spring)
spread her wings and pump the April into them
to mark the end of March.

You would have known more about so many things
if you hadn't whooped and danced and shook your fists
as the chrysalis broke and gold wet wings appeared.

(Published in *Off the Coast*)

Mr. Pain

∼ The pain is bad today; it breaks through the Oxycodone. My throat has closed some more, and what I'm able to drink makes me gag. J tries to cheer me up.

"Maybe you should try the smart version of that drug."

"Huh?"

"You know, Foxycodone."

She groans, but I'm already groaning louder.

"Or the one where the pill is in the shape of a cube."

"I give up."

"Boxycodone."

A few minutes pass. "You know they make a dosage of that stuff that gives strippers extra courage."

"What?"

"Roxy Moxycodone."

Good try, not much help. It's a bad day for prose (as you can probably tell). Lemme try the other form:

Mr. Pain

Mr. Pain is a gentleman,
a scientist, a writer of prose.
He doesn't wake me, he stands
Respectfully beside my bed

Mr. Pain

His glowing steel fingers politely
tucked beneath cactus spine arms.

He waits 'til I'm awake, 'til I know
that I'm not in my dream but in this bed.
He watches my eyes, listens for my breath
And he reaches for my face
To begin his grim undertaking.

Mr. Pain is head technician
In this raw neural laboratory.
He welcomes me back
From the night's rest and into
The day's dark research.

(Published in *Out of Our* in 2012)

Aspiration

〰️ By a little trick of the English language, *aspiration* means both "something devoutly wished for" and "the act of removing fluid from a cavity of the body by inserting a hollow needle." You can "cherish" an aspiration or you can "undergo" one, but you don't get to choose.

• • •

Yesterday's scheduled punch biopsy turned into the more elegant-sounding fine needle aspiration. I've never cherished any sort of needle aspiration, much less a fine one.

What they do is the opposite of an injection. They stick the needle in your skin, and then they pull the plunger on the syringe out to extract a piece (actually, some small pieces) of you. The cytology lab will examine those cells, taken from the sore and swollen lump under my jaw, to see if it's cancerous. It hurts, maybe a six or seven on the pain scale. The typical draw is three separate shots. With three samples, they're sure that they got some of the right cells. The surgeon does the first one, and then he asks me if I can stand two more. Do I have a choice? Well, the lab likes three samples, but he figures he's good enough to get it in one or two. I turn my head away, and he does it again. (I'm squeezing J's hand, fortunately too weak to do any damage.)

Aspiration

It's mostly fluid, but he can see cells floating around. Off to the lab to see if the cells are cancer.

. . .

The test takes two days, but they'll let me know in a week. Why the delay? One thought is that the patient is better off getting bad news if there's a doctor around when it's delivered. I wonder how my doctors would feel if I knew something that was vital to their well-being and I was planning on telling them four days from now.

Would they feel patronized? Just wondering.

A Very Cruel Thing to Do to Sick People

∼ I'm thin and weak, and I don't eat very much. Maybe it's because I'm nauseated all the time. I'm certainly dehydrated, because it hurts so much to drink that it's easier to stay thirsty. The docs are sending me for a dose of intravenous anti-nausea drug. There's a room at Fox Chase that's devoted to "infusing." It's also where you get chemotherapy. My appointment is at 11:00.

Three hours later, I'm still waiting for my name to be called. I haven't eaten, and the pain meds have worn off. The lump under my jaw is throbbing. Worse yet, there are people there with the awful gray tint of chemo on them slumped into upright chairs or sliding out of wheelchairs and staring off at something that I can't see right now. They're suffering.

In circumstances like these, I'm usually pretty polite. I know that the young woman behind the counter isn't the one responsible for scheduling more people than the infusion room can hold. But I gotta say something, and here's what I say, whispering:

"Hi. I hate to bother you, and I know it's not your fault, but it's been three hours now since my appointment. This is a very cruel thing to do to sick people."

All I'm looking for is a nod, and I get one. I guess she knows. Fifteen minutes later they call me in.

• • •

The anti-nausea drug—Kytril—didn't work, and at midnight, I'm standing in the bathroom, retching and musing.

"Non-diagnostic"

That's how the surgeon describes the results of my fine needle aspiration biopsy. I am so taken by the sheer ambition of the phrase that it's going to be my new expression, the cliché by which ye shall know me.

It means "I have no idea what the results of that painful and expensive test indicate, and I hope if I talk fast enough and change the subject, no one will ask me why I ordered it in the first place."

A bit more conversation in which it becomes clear that nobody has any good ideas about why I'm still feeling lousy and losing weight. Learned physicians look away and mumble when I ask about the source of the pain, which is now so constant and intense that I wake up in the middle of the night to take dope. And then we wait until the seventh of February for another scan and another week for results. In the meantime, I'm going to the dentist and officially offering myself up as quack-bait. Crystals? Vibrations? Can I sleep in your pyramid?

• • •

The dentist shoots me up with Novocain, and the pain in my jaw disappears. So the good news is that part of my pain comes from a mere toothache. The bad news is that I have a root canal in my near future.

Do Root Canals Cure Cancer?

∿ The root canal is set for Monday at 11:00. In the meantime, the snow is melting in Carpenter's Woods.

january after the snow

carpenter's woods

last week the white grayed down
little yellow caverns melted in and refrozen.
little turds—the punctuation
of brown gems flush—set in the crust
of last week's snow.
and there was a wash of gray
just because the snow lives here
under the same dirty roof as us.

last week the woods wanted to tell us
that every drift has its own shit
and any warmth will soften the deepest chill
and that every day has its gray.

this week, a thaw:
you won't see a lump or sump
beside the trails in carpenter's woods.

Do Root Canals Cure Cancer?

today the woods will tell us
that it's got enough earth
to cover a multitude
and there's no harm that won't disappear
in sweet decay and earth and time.

Instead of a Root Canal . . .

. . . we end up in the triage unit at Fox Chase. I woke up weak and dizzy and fainting. Those didn't seem like qualifications you'd bring to two hours of dental surgery, so J drove me in. Five hours later, infused with saline and loaded with an anti-nausea drug called Aloxi, we left.

I'm weak and dehydrated, not getting enough nourishment—hell, I've hardly been nourished at all. I weigh 135 pounds, and I've pretty much forgotten what it's like to chew, swallow, or feel warm.

The current wisdom is that I get infused once a day. The infusion is a liter of saline solution, hung on a pole and dripped through a tube into my port. Otherwise, I have to force food and drink and... what? Well, nobody knows.

PET Scans and Michael Douglas

~ A PET scan is a look at your body's processes, not its structures. It takes some particular function like blood flow or oxygen use and shows the degree to which it's occurring in various parts of the body. So if you know that cancerous tissue uses glucose at a higher rate than normal tissue, you can spot the cancer by injecting radioactive glucose into a hungry person and then seeing where the radiation—and therefore the glucose uptake—is most intense.

This is the granddaddy of diagnostic tests. It's the one that should tell them definitively if all that treatment worked or didn't. We've been through this before: scans and biopsies. I've become so used to inconclusive answers that I'm almost numb to the results. You're gonna tell me if it's life or death? Yeah, buddy, right.

From the patient's point of view, the whole thing is pretty uneventful, except for the requirement that you fast for four hours before the test. If your scan is at 10:00 a.m., let's say, that means that you probably will have been foodless for twelve hours or so. Then you get a relatively painless shot (she only missed the vein once) and wait for an hour. So, there I was, at 11:30, wobbly and dizzy and waiting. I pretended I had a moderate buzz. I think I meditated; maybe I just slept.

The hard part for us head-and-neck types is that you have to lie on your back without moving for the duration of the scan—a

PET Scans and Michael Douglas

half hour or so. If you're an Artesian well for phlegm—as we tend to be—that's hard to do without choking. After a bit of panic, we figured out that a slight elevation of the head kept the stuff from backing up. That done, the procedure is a snap, and the wooziness is almost a help getting through it.

Someone will have the results in a day or two, and as soon as they trickle down to me, I'll let you know.

• • •

Maybe you saw the Super Bowl halftime show. It started with a photo of Michael Douglas (he's the other celebrity head-and-neck cancer guy). He narrated a little something about rising to the challenges, 9/11, and, oh, Valley Forge and the Battle of the Bulge. Two people got in touch to say how inspired they were. What nobody mentioned is that the picture of Douglas is a still, a file shot presumably from happier times. I'm assuming that's because he may still be a bit withered from treatment, sort of like me. I'm also assuming that he's on his way to recovery but not quite ready to take the full show on the road. Just like me.

• • •

I am cold. I dress to keep the warmth in, layers and layers, like putting the fat back on my body, but it really doesn't work. I went to bed last night wearing a hat and socks and long underwear, and I shivered.

J introduces me to fleece. Not the sheepish kind and certainly not the golden one. This is fabric made from old plastic toe-tags or some such and sewn (molded?) into garments. It's ugly and it's warm. I'm a fan.

Bad News and New Tires

∾ I've become used to it: there's a test—a scan, a scrape, a scope. We wait for a few days or a week, and then they say the test was inconclusive. "Getting test results" is now an item on a checklist, below "getting groceries" and above "dry cleaning."

Today, on the way to Fox Chase to hear the results of the last scan, I dropped off a tire to be replaced—son of a gun jumped right off its rim—and checked in to the clinic.

This PET scan was not inconclusive, my oncologist says. I am not unsurprised, and I hope that you will be unbored to hear it. It showed something growing right where the tumor was. What is it? It's probably a tumor, no, it's probably *the* tumor. There are a few reasons to think that it might be just inflammation, but nobody seemed very convinced. I was getting better, and now the symptoms are getting worse. The smart money is all on tumor redux.

Here's what's next. I meet with the surgeon on Friday, and we schedule—you guessed it—another surgical look around. Depending on what he sees, he'll develop a plan for surgery to remove it. This is complicated business, involving reconstructive surgeons and other specialists. Think D-Day or *Spider-Man*, the musical.

On the way home, I picked up the tire, shiny and smelly on its rim. J tells me that I didn't do the right thing (the new tire should be on the car, not in the trunk), but my judgment on automotive matters has never been too good. I don't think I'll worry about it much right now.

On Delivering Bad News

～ Back in August, a person whose scope had just been down my throat said flatly, "It's cancer." It was the first time the word had been mentioned, and it opened a hole in the floor through which I fell into Cancerland. Both J and I had to blink. Did she really say that? Did she really let us hear how little she cared? Doesn't even the sentencing judge lower her voice and ask for someone to have mercy on something?

Today, Dr. Barbara Burtness, my oncologist, opened up a blank in the conversation and let me fill it. When she walked in the examining room, she was quiet; I could feel her reluctance to speak, and, to make it easier for both of us, I guessed what had to be so. Bad news, eh?

Of course, in the past few months, I've gotten used to cancer, come to expect it to be around. The difference between these two announcements has nothing to do with my familiarity, however. The difference was that this time the doctor cared.

For those of you who have to deliver bad news from time to time, here's the secret. What you have to do is open yourself up—even if just for a minute—to the sense that the news is bad and that someone's going to be hurt. Allow that, in an obscenely tiny way, the giant spear through the heart is going to splash some blood on you, too. Let yourself feel it. Chances are that those of us who are about to die have already guessed what's up. And for making it easier for both of us, we salute you.

If you can't quite bring yourself to do that, I guess it's up to us to help you out.

Conclusive Results

~ Now we're getting conclusive—as in conclusion, as in coming to an end. Dr. Ridge, lean and resonant like a giant bass violin, tells me that it's a tumor—almost certainly. Unfortunately, he can't really see the thing from the picture, so he has to go in and take a closer look. He knows it's big, has to see how big, so tomorrow there's yet another biopsy.

Draw the bow one more time. Once he sees what's there, he'll be able to make plans for what's called a resection. They break through the lower jaw and open it up like a book. Then they remove the tumor.

If they get it all, we start a period of rehab—about eighteen months. Rebuilding jaws, re-muscle-ing tongues. It doesn't actually return to normal, but it improves. If they don't get it, well, it's cancer, and cancer, my dears, has its own program. Overall, how does it look? ("What's my chance, doc? Give it to me straight.")

There are two answers to that question.

Dr. Ridge's answer is, "Most people in your situation die."

My answer? "But not me, baby." There are books to write, a kid to see through law school, a dog to walk, a fine and ripe old love to polish. There's no way I'm going to die—choking and starving—before I hit seventy. Besides, who wants to read about that?

But there's something else: most people die? Yes, no, actually, all people die. So all those things I want to do and feel, they've got

117

to happen now. Death is your friend; he tells you to be alive. Now. I really don't need some doctor who turns my head away from that or mushes it all up with hope. I need someone to remind me that time is short or that even if it's long, it's limited. So, really, it's "Yes, me, too. I'm gonna die, but I'm gonna whoop my cancerous self up for as long as I got. Thanks, Doc."***

I'm almost weepingly grateful to him, imagine how daring it is to put up a truthful sign-post in a wilderness of banal nonsense.

** A few months later, Dr. Ridge hears that I'm referring to him as Dr. Death. Surprisingly, he gets huffy about it. Go figure.

More Conclusive

〜 My friend Jamie (who writes under the name J. R. Lankford) probably has a secret doctorate in applied symbology†† or something like it. She asked me a few days ago if I could use a sword or a steed as I made my way through the cancer wars.

Today a box arrived with six miniature T'ang dynasty horses "to help me do battle."

The horsies must have helped, because when I swam up from the bottom of the anesthetic late this afternoon, the surgeon said that whatever is clogging up my throat didn't look like cancer to him. There's still a pathologist who has to gape at the scrapings, but he's pretty sure. I'm believing him for two reasons. First of all, he sounded like a man who was happy to be playing this particular solo recitation: "You Live, You Live!" by Dr. Drew Ridge. Second, I'm believing it because I want to believe it. I live.

So, it looks like my next job is getting healthy—more on that tomorrow when the fog lifts.

• • •

Two other things I want to tell you before I go to sleep:

---

†† She once wrote a thriller called *The Jesus Thief* that keeps you on the edge of your chair, even though it's also quite clearly a retelling of the fairly well-known Jesus myth. You do know that story, don't you? Suffering, resurrection, and so on . . .

RADIATION DAYS

1. Tonight, around 10:05, I cried for about fifteen seconds, and then I laughed for maybe ten, and then the whole hot thing chilled and became a tiny spinning mirror out in front of me somewhere.
2. The song that's planted itself in my brain is a fragment from "Hallelujah, I'm a Bum." The song goes on:

> Hallelujah, I'm a bum
> Hallelujah bum again
> Hallelujah, gimme a bum bum
> To revive us again

What the hell do you make of that?

Unrequited Love—Part One

～ I've had a long relationship with wine and beer. About thirty years ago, when beer was just beginning to make the cultural leap from Working-Class Alcohol Conveyor to Object Worthy of Gourmet Veneration, I was under contract to write a book that would introduce people to the lore and the pleasure of beer. That book never made it to stores, but a few years ago, a modern version did. It was called the *Short Course in Beer*. The *Short Course in Beer*, like me, got a second chance and a second edition.

Short Course gave me the chance to acknowledge my admiration for one of life's under-recognized delights. A few years before the beer book came out, I published a textbook about wine with a company called Prentice Hall. It was called *The New Short Course in Wine*.

When I lead tastings, people often look at the little stacks of books and ask, "So, what do you like better, wine or beer?" Of course, I'd much rather they asked something like, "Do you have a couple of extra cases of these?" or "Is it too late to bid on the movie rights?"

When I feel like taking the question seriously, I say something like, "I love beer, but I need red wine." (Yup, just red.) I explain that a delicious, well-composed beer is a thing of great beauty, maybe even a thing unrivaled in the world of tasting for its sheer ability to deliver the flavor. But when the moment is emotionally important—when it transcends matters of taste or mere sensation—I need the solemnity, the organ-blasting, choir-of-angels effect of a good glass of red. I'm not talking necessarily about highlights film stuff here. If I hadn't seen you in while and I bumped into you crossing Rittenhouse Square, for instance, there's no question that we would mark the moment with red wine. The funny thing is that the wine for an occasion doesn't have to be great in itself; it's really just enough that it be red and decently made and in a glass.

Beer is beautiful, but red's a sacrament.

Last night, I decided to have a glass just to acknowledge that one out of one doctors say that I might live through this damn thing. The wine was the beautiful Piazza della Torre made by the equally beautiful Marilisa Allegrini. The bouquet is a concentrated fruit blast with the unmistakable raisin-y intensity of a Ripasso wine. And the first sip! Ah. It's like inviting that whole orchestra into your mouth to jam. But in this case, the orchestra started stripping the wallpaper off the walls and trashing the room.

Right. The fragile layer of moisture in my mouth was burned away, and the crackling, shrinking, sere sensation of fragile membrane folding and drying and blistering took over. Just enough time to dive for the Ensure to put out the fire.

The villain, of course, is my old friend Tannin, the wonderful phenol that puts the dry in and takes all the other tastes out. But chemistry be damned, what's happened is that one of my ritual anchors doesn't hold bottom any more.

What happens now? Dismay? Depression? Sudden Enlightenment? I'll let you know.

There's No Evidence

～ Dr. Ridge is in a hurry today. He hasn't sat down when he says, "There's no evidence of cancer." From there on I don't remember much. I know he trimmed his sails a bit, said something about *no evidence not being the same as no cancer*. There was also something about radiation and eighteen months to recover, and there was definitely a "see you later" in there. And now it's my daughter's birthday, and if you'll excuse me . . .

How to Prevent Throat Cancer in Two Parts

Part One

The most important thing to know about preventing throat cancer is this: you can't prevent throat cancer.

What you can do is reduce your chances of getting it by taking a few simple, if horrifying steps. First of all, don't smoke. There are thousands of reasons to avoid smoking, most of which contain the word "cancer" or refer to some other loathsome disease. If you had to wait to think about preventing throat cancer before you thought about quitting smoking, you just haven't been paying very close attention.

RADIATION DAYS

Tobacco smoking is so vile that it really doesn't take the threat of throat cancer to make it an eminently quittable practice. If you smoke, you smell. No, that's too polite—you stink. People edge away from you; they suggest meeting by telephone instead of for lunch. They prefer to see you outdoors—in winter. You find that you get some interesting propositions for phone sex (from people who have been your lover for years). When you meet a friend on the street, they always move to your upwind side. Your dry cleaner handles your clothes with tongs.

There are jobs you can't get, relationships you can't have, and airplane flights that are torture to you. What do you get in return? Well, you get an addiction that makes you wheeze, stink, and run out of breath at the top of a short flight of stairs. You get an addiction that just about guarantees an early death from a disgusting and painful disease (the folks with the heart attacks are the lucky ones).

The easiest way to quit smoking is to get cancer. No doubt about it, the simple words "you've got cancer" are the greatest magic spell to dissolve the long, romantic, very personal bond you have with smoking. All of a sudden your brand, your rituals, your paraphernalia, even your grandfather's Zippo lighter with the word FLORSHEIM engraved on the brushed steel case will lose their appeal in a second. Nobody walks out on the Bad Diagnosis and lights up one last one for old time's sake.

Perhaps you'd prefer a less radical approach. What worked for me was having a baby. That, and SmokEnders and Valium and exercising two hours a day and eating entire chickens in one sitting and washing them down with full bottles of Zinfandel. I also had to be willing to sacrifice several friendships with people who could no longer stand to be around the hyper-irritable tinderbox that I became. It only took about nine months, and if you've got the time and the womb, it's not a bad way to go. The best thing about this approach is that at the end, you're smoke-free and you get to keep the kid.

There are even easier ways, but I don't know much about them. What matters is this: if you want to prevent throat cancer, you don't have a prayer until you stop smoking.

Part Two

One of the things you can do to lower your risk is exercise. I haven't seen any explanations, but the consistent observation is that the virtuous exercisers—the lean-butt, flat-ab, snaky-triceps crowd—are less likely to come down with cancer.

Of course, it's a little too late for me, but one of the pieces that goes along with good health is being active, so today I started walking. My friend Gilmore talked me into it. On a mild, spring-ish day, he dragged me out of the house for a mile and a half around the track. Part prevention, part restoration.

I came home, didn't pass out, ate everything in sight that was mushy enough to get down, and while I can't say that I feel better, I do feel virtuous.

Restoration Software

~ Treating cancer with radiation therapy and chemotherapy is a bit like treating the dog for fleas by setting him on fire. You may very well get rid of the bugs, but when the flames die down, you're going to have a severely damaged dog on your hands.

Assuming that they really did get all my cancer, the pup they left behind is—by most common measures—in pretty bad shape. I've lost about forty-five pounds of body weight, and I look skeletal. I can't really chew, and it's hard to swallow anything but bland, milky liquids. Most foods just turn into clay in my mouth, and a lot of liquids hurt. Old friends like wine and beer are painful, tea gives a hurtful dryness, and fruit juice burns.

Being undernourished means that I'm also weak. A trip to the gym shows a strength loss of about 50 percent in most muscle groups.

I still have a lot of pain in my throat and neck, so I'm still a regular user of painkillers, which, aside from promoting ten to twelve hours of sleep a day, have a host of other charming side effects. I'll spare you the details, except to say that one of them rhymes with "inspiration." I don't have much energy, and while I might be fending off depression, a serious case of the glooms could happen any time.

So, it's time to make a plan, develop my own Restoration Software.

This week I'm consulting with all my doctors and with some new therapists. There's one for speech and even one who specializes in teaching you how to swallow. Yes, I'll be doing swallowing exercises. I'm also heading back to the gym on a five-day-a-week schedule and reducing my painkillers. I don't know what I can do about my lousy eating habits—I can't really chew and swallow anything that needs serious chewing—except for setting a goal of 2,000 calories a day and seeing how much Ensure one man can gulp down.

I'm glad I have my new teaching assignment; it's given me a stack of reading and a ton of thinking to do. I have some lectures to write, and there are two novels that could use some attention—maybe that will be enough to beat back depression. Even though there's some danger of a backfire, I want to take on a self-education project and become a bit more web-competent.

Anyway, that's my Restoration Software. I'll keep you posted on the output.

Vitamin Sleep or...Rest Ye Merry

～ Here's a little recovery tip. You can share it with your post-radiation treatment friends.

Radiation makes you tired. Doesn't matter where you got irradiated, asshole or elbow, radiation robs you of energy, and the effect lasts for months. It's a mean-ass, ugly fatigue, the sort of thing that comes up on you while you're in the middle of page 112 and smacks you down so hard that you wake up two hours later with your thumb still on the same page. Even with Dr. Dry Mouth (xerostomia) waking you up every hour or two at night, this is fatigue that's always glad to welcome you back.

What should you do about a world-class case of the flopsies? Rest. Take it easy and don't, I say, brothers and sisters, don't blame yourself. It's your body paying the price for the radiation that killed the cancer. There is a nasty puritanism about in our culture that will allow you any symptom of illness except fatigue. If you have to sleep ten hours a night, the little puritan says, there's something wrong with you. Not something wrong with your body, but with your soul. "*No giving in!*" it shouts. (How come these preachers are always shouting?) Well, if you run into that nasty puritan, tell him that you're tired of him. In fact, tell him to get out of your life, that rest is the first part of rest(oration) and that you may be sick, but you know when to let sleeping cancer patients lie.

If the nasty little bastard is somebody close to you, be sure to establish firm boundaries. You know when you're tired, just like you know when you're hungry and you know when you're horny. No discussion required. In fact you are the World's Foremost Authority on your sleep needs. It's not a moral issue; it's medical, and you're the doctor. Period.

And if the puritan in question is you? I guess it depends on how you talk to yourself, but the message is the same. Don't beat yourself up, just lay yourself down.

It will get better, at least that's what they tell me.

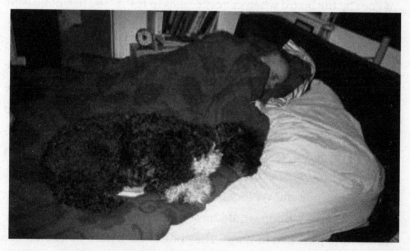

You'll have to get your own dog. Photo by Dr. Brigitte Steger

Stay Awake and Socialize

〜 You may have wondered what a nauseated, sleepy, emaci-
ated person does for a social life. Well, mostly he answers email.
Occasionally, to spice things up, he may send a text. But the old-
fashioned, soul-in-a-room-of-other-souls kind of hobnobbing kind
of goes by the board when cancer comes to town. The hermetic gene
starts expressing itself, and you really don't get out much anymore.

Next week, I'm teaching two classes. There's a beer tasting in
Mt. Airy (Trappist Ales) and a lecture on Gastronomy and Culture
at Atlantic Cape CC. Aside from the demands on stamina, I'll have
to revive whatever social skills I once faked and remember how to
be with groups of people again.

So, my good fortune this week is to have two nights out. Last
night, I sat in on Andrew Gilmore's seminar on cartoons from the
pre–Hayes Code era. We looked at Betty Boop and Popeye. (Actually,
we sort of ogled. Boop would have seduced Charlie Sheen; Popeye
would have punched him out. They both would have done it for the
sheer fun of the thing. Andrew is as quietly entertaining as Boop
is outrageous.)

Tonight, our neighbors Harry and Sara declared the First Night
of Porch Season. It's a very big deal here in Philadelphia, so we sidled
on over with snacks and a winter-full of repressed neighborly conversation. I brought a growler of homemade beer—a Saison that I

130

brewed before the nasty diagnosis. The batch has been untouched for about eight months and sitting quietly thinking about itself in J's cool cellar. It was copper-colored with a passable head and a spicy-earthy nose. In the mouth, well—in my mouth—it was clean and rich with a slightly toasted, full-on malt presence and a crisp, mouth-watering finish. You could smell the pilsner malt and the tad of biscuit that went into it. Very easy to drink.

Wait. Did I say *easy to drink*? It wasn't too long ago that bubbles and acidity hurt my mouth. In fact, what with chewing being so difficult these days, it was easy enough to drink dinner. My neighbors thought so, too, and we ended up drinking two 2-liter growlers: one refrigerated, the other at cellar temperature. Nobody complained about warm beer, no one thought the color was odd, and a few folks thought that they might want to brew something themselves.

So, now, for next week I have stirred up some images. I can tell people about how Social Structure (the code) affects Culture (the cartoon). I can use that as a foil to talk about how Napoleon's spanking the monasteries ultimately led to Trappist Ale. That may lead me to talk about the cute little way we have of letting ourselves slide back and forth between different meanings of the same word without even noticing. (I was going to use a trombone to illustrate the point, but Betty Boop is Better. I mean better.)

Then I also have the example of a bunch of people on a twilight porch drinking a very unconventionally colored and flavored beer. with the lights almost out, there was only the flavor, and the flavor made friends.

Damn, it's good to get out.

Two Visitors

〜 Friday, in Carpenter's Woods, I saw two butterflies—my first of the year. One was a startling, high-speed, crazy-energized Hackberry Emperor. I had to stand still while it dive-bombed the little patch of sunlight, lit on a downed tree, and took off again. It was minutes, or maybe even a lifetime until it slowed up enough for me to see what it was. The other was a Mourning Cloak, so dark brown it was black. It would have been invisible but for its little jaunt into the sun to dry out its wings.

I was so grateful to see them; they reminded me what there is to lose of this world. Nothing like it in winter.

Restoration Interrupted/ Life Summary—Part Five

So with Imagination (and maybe a touch of Depression)
the butterflies turn in to emblems to sew just so.
I'll wear one per shoulder.
Maybe emblems of my two granddaddy flaws,
the ones that have caused me the most tumult, the most sorrow,
the strongest smell of life half-lived, of luscious crumbs
left on the plate to delight the dishwasher and feed the drain.
They are Fear and Laziness, these granddaddy badges.

We'll let the Mourning Cloak be Fear and what's to fear now?
I can't lose the lost, I died just a while back. It's fine.
My Passover passed over, this cat-on-lap afternoon a bonus.
But the Hackberry Emperor, ah! Call him Laziness!
Him of the heavy limbs, and fatted lids.
Fear's little brother with the cuddly slippers and the shades pulled down.
Tiny beats of tawny wings. Little marriage-killer, book-spurner,
flabbifier, sure to try her.
He'll keep me in today.
It's raining and it's cold outside and besides
it's way too late.

Tomorrow, there's another pupa poppin'
Another scaly eclosed thing.
Let's see, let's see
What the butterflies bring.

RADIATION DAYS

And will we rise
Or will we not
At the sight of the
Slivery Checkerspot?

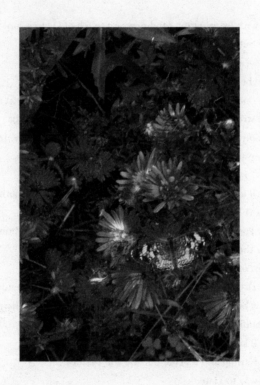

Grown-Up Food

~ Mostly these days, it's mush for me. I blend up some cereal with milk and a few berries; I eat cottage cheese and clam chowder, applesauce, ice cream, oatmeal, stuff like that. I try not to think of it as pre-chewed food, but that's the general idea: anything I eat has to come with its own saliva, 'cause I'm fresh out.

Soft foods have a certain infantile air about them. (In fact, I've looked the baby food aisle over once or twice.) I don't mind; eating mush beats the hell out of not eating at all.

But the one grown-up food that I can chew is sashimi. The fish is soft and moist, and the flavors—in a good sushi restaurant—can be superb. As it happens, I live about forty minutes away from one of the best sushi restaurants in the country. I once spent a month in Japan and never found anything like it. It's Chefs Jesse and Matt Ito's magnificent Fuji, and it's located on the main street in Haddonfield, a little exurb over in Jersey. Tonight, J and I decided that it was time that I started eating like a grown-up, even if I'm not too chew-ish.

I won't take you through the whole meal; let's just say it was like getting one of my senses restored. Without too much jaw fatigue or dry mouth, we worked through eight different kinds of sushi, including a live scallop drizzled with truffle oil (surf and turf) that I'll probably remember forever for its leaping, vaulting oceanic

135

finish and a lightly marinated salmon that was so good we had to have seconds. For a man who's been living mostly on semi-digested human chow, the dance of tastes was thrilling, dramatic—a night at the opera and a day at the beach.

The best thing was the course that was thrown in. We didn't ask, but chef knew about my situation and dropped this in front of us:

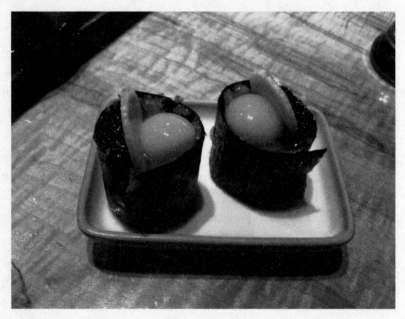

The yolks are from quails' eggs; the black, shiny stuff is caviar.

You say you can't stand the thought of eating a raw egg? Great, just pass yours over here.

Finding My Voice Again

～ I started today. I got in the car and drove fifty-five miles to Atlantic Cape Culinary Academy. I filled out the paperwork that would permit me to be paid, found my cubicle, printed out my notes, swallowed coffee, walked to my classroom, said hello, and started talking.

What am I talking about? That's always a good question. People, including me, ask it all the time. Today, I was talking about making sense of a college course called Culture and Gastronomy. Here's an excerpt from my lecture notes:

> So, let's get back to Gastronomy and Culture—I'm intimidated by the words myself. One word sounds pretty pompous; the other has so many meanings that we can slip among them without noticing that we've changed what we're talking about.

And, yes, I have to admit that I'm slipping around here, too. I decided to focus on what they're calling Modernist Cuisine because I've wondered for a long time how Modernism: The Trend affected Modernism: The Fashion in Food. In fact, I've wondered for years about food's position as a weird outlier in the world of Fashion. We can go naked, but we can't go hungry, and food swings—or does it rotate?—in long arcs of High Fashion and Low. The rise and fall, I mean the Rise and Fall of the Tastykake completely underlapping the Rise and Fall of Cuisine Minceur. Can this mean anything? Is it just trivial, or is something hiding? I want to know, just because I want to. It's not necessary to me; I can love the food I cook and the food I eat and it doesn't have to mean anything. I can be happy that it makes me and us happy, that we camp on the side of the angels when we cook beautifully and eat well.

But now, I've got to put up or shut up.

Gordon Bowles and Ageya Bharati are watching you, man.

There are nine students at one of the best culinary schools in the country sitting in front of me with notebooks open. I know a lot of stuff, but do I know what I'm talking about? The only way I'm going to find out is to start talking and see what comes out of my mouth. Is this fair to them? Well, I've had a lot of courses where the professor put out all she knew and didn't even take a crack at the big questions. Some of those courses were the best ones of my life, but I'm aiming for something better. After all, this is a comeback, and there ought to be something good to come back to. Something good to come back to.

Francis O'Laughlin at Hobart College—say the name and tremble before you walk in a classroom, boy.

At least, I should know what the terms mean. Here's what my notes have for Modern:

> *Modern* means a significant break with the past founded on new or newly diffused knowledge and/or new moral perspective.
>
> I'm sure someone has this better, but it's what I'm working with today. It's a backwards definition, one I built by starting with what I know about modern cooking and going backwards. Fair enough.

Then there's culture. I've got my anthro-pants down around my knees here. I remember pages of "definitions" and seminars of circular discussions. "What's culture?" "It's X and Y and Z." "OK, but what about B and R?" "Oh, yeah, that, too." So, I know the important thing with a definition here is the *fini* part. You gotta stop somewhere. I stop like this:

> *Culture* is human nature as processed by humans. Cathedrals and cartwheels, ways of talking, and the grammar of walking. Let's assume that a person can participate in more than one culture and that cultures can be large and inclusive (Han Chinese) or small and particular (Bolivian soccer fans).
>
> Let's allow that culture is usually passed from parents to children, but that transmission isn't perfect. We have whisper-down-the-lane rather than digital duplication. Because of that, cultures change. They change because of duplication drift (you ain't your daddy) and also because cultures meet when peoples meet. Sometimes when cultures meet, you get a mash-up: characteristics thrown together like in red-bean ice cream. Sometimes (more often) you get genuinely new products: spaghetti and meatballs. The term for this is *syncretism* (note slightly different use in philosophy).

Then, worst of all is gastronomy.

All of this brings us to our working definition of *gastronomy*:

The food that mom would have made if she had the time, money, energy, information, and community support to do so.

Let's take a minute with that "if." If there isn't enough food to go around, or if there are only a few kinds of food, there's no gastronomy. Gastronomy depends on abundance and variety. Without abundance, there's no creative struggle; there's just struggle. That's the first characteristic of gastronomy. Second: there is a value attached to food beyond nutrition. Third: that value itself can be the subject of discussion. Fourth: gastronomy is about food that we have transformed. This is key.

RADIATION DAYS

So I go on from there: culture is cooking, ya see. Why do we cook at all? Who are we anyway? Claude, Levi, and Strauss. Do I know what I'm talking about? Well, yeah, I've spent a lot of time with this stuff. Is my knowing about it going to take these students someplace new?

As we say in Cancerland: stay tuned.

Right there in the front row, Smith, Baptiste, and McClay have their notebooks open. Nyheim and McFadden are all ears. Gotta get it right.

The Gala

～ There's a fringe benefit with my new job. I got to go to a black-tie bash at Bally's Casino in Atlantic City. It's a benefit for the Academy of Culinary Arts, and about one million people show up, pay $200 a pop, and eat and drink and dance in their fancies all night long.

My job was to hob and nob—and I did my best with swollen tongue and clenched throat. It was easier when I wasn't pretending that I could eat like a normal person and just swigged my Ensure. It's easier then to obey the rule about not talking with your mouth full, because in my condition, if you're trying to eat solid food, your mouth is never truly empty.

Aside from the students, who are just adorable, and my colleagues, who work so hard and with such grace, the best part of the evening was my hotel room. Good ol' 2730. It was big with windows facing the ocean and looking north along the beach toward New York. The view from the bathtub was great, the view from the living room even better (if you reversed the chairs so they were facing toward instead of away from the ocean).

My new dream home may be an apartment in Atlantic City with a window facing east.

In fact, it was hard for me to move away from it. I checked in early, figuring I could walk around, dig the boardwalk, maybe start an argument with a gull, or goddamn a clam. Something salty like that. But I found I couldn't leave the room. For about two hours before and maybe three hours after, I sat and stared out the window. Even the thought of gorgeous women in evening gowns didn't break in to the trance. I remember that toward midnight, I started singing myself a song, trying to soothe something, some screaming meemee that was threatening to burst its way up from beneath the calm, I guess.

Here it is, as well as I can remember it on Saturday:

Dolly Parton and her brother Martin
Just can't seem to stop from startin'
smokin' fish and catchin' joints
and winning games by elebenty points.

And How ARE You?

~ A friend who's just lost his job and is throwing a party to celebrate writes, "So how ARE you? (I figure this will save you talking at the party . . .)"

I'm glad he asked.

I'm sort of like a guy all dressed up in black tie, standing at the dessert table all by himself—without a sweet tooth to his name. You say that doesn't help?

OK, I feel pretty good. I still have damage from the radio and chemo. My mouth is dry a lot; I'm still eating mostly mush. I get occasional sharp pains, like the ones that led to the discovery of the cancer. My tongue is swollen, and I don't recognize my own voice. I don't know for sure if I'm free of cancer because the scans show something there—could be malignant, could be scar tissue.

I can't eat regular food, can't abide wine in my mouth. I'm weak, tired, and looking like the guy who could play the role of Death in the annual morality pageant.

I've got a new temporary job. The people are lovely, and the task is doable (Culture and Gastronomy: the Rise of Modernism), five lectures plus a wine tasting, a beer tasting, and a lecture to the faculty. It's really good to be back at that again; teaching is still my favorite thing of things.

So, I'm like a guy with a reprieve and on parole. I am enjoying 'most every day, carpe-ing each diem as it comes along. Not exactly well, but I think this is what happy feels like. Sort of. There's still a few wishes I'd like to have granted, but being in wish isn't the same as being in want.

The funny thing is that I've never had such a complete answer to that question in my life. Funny what cancer can do for you and now that you mention it: how are you?

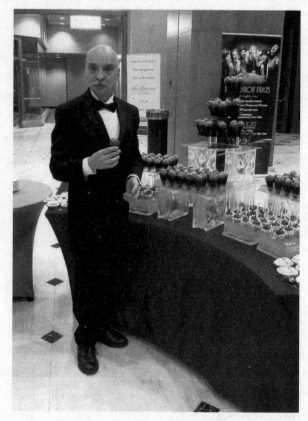

How AM I? Sort of like this.

Root Canal

∾ It's time to get it over with. I didn't exactly get myself admitted to the hospital to avoid a root canal, but it was a good excuse for putting it off. The dentist is out in the suburbs someplace, and he's got Phillies tickets for the night game. The root canal is interrupted twice by phone calls from his friends. They're sitting third base–side, "looking right in on the right-handed pitchers." I'm glad to hear it. In spite of the chat, and because of the nitrous oxide, the whole thing is over in thirty-five easy minutes. The nurse worries that the nitrous level may be too high. I tell her I'm an old hippie and she shouldn't worry. By the time I get back to J's, the anesthetic has worn off, and by bedtime, I've forgotten that it happened.

Restoring the Strength and Resorting to Addiction

Addiction

Addiction is the Messenger Cow
Thank it, Kill it, Eat it. Now
Pan-sear with Mushrooms
Deglaze with stock.
Anoint your eyes, your heart, your cock.
It's a john-the-baptist, A Bachelor's Cat.
Addiction tells us where we're at.
Clean your plate and wipe your chin,
When the Cow is gone, just look within.

• • •

∼ Three weeks ago, J bought me a gym membership. It was time.

About twenty-four years ago, I stopped smoking. I didn't leave Smokeland gracefully. In fact, I was one of the most miserable, irritable sons of bitches you'd ever run into in your life. I could start an argument with your collar button. It's amazing that, during the nine months of really bad withdrawal, no one shot or divorced me. One of the things that got me through was a gym on top of a high-rise in Center City Philadelphia. I walked there every day, and for about two hours, I lifted weights and swam until I was exhausted.

Restoring the Strength and Resorting to Addiction

For those hours, and maybe one hour afterward, I didn't have that explosive, vitriolic craving for a cigarette. Maybe three hours a day, I could stand the company of the person I was without nicotine. In the way these things happen, the exertion came to be a kind of drug for me. Somewhere in the exhaustion of doing one more repetition of an exercise, one more than my body really wanted to do, my brain cracked and something wonderful leaked out. To call it substituting one addiction for another probably misses the point, but it isn't wrong, either. Short story: over all those twenty-four years, my self came to include this regular brain-breaking dance with the weights. Picking up heavy things until I disappeared inside the effort became my hobby, my Tao, and the gym, any gym, was my dojo. Wanna know how serious I was? My six-year-old daughter named her new puppy Muscular. That's serious. That's love.

Then cancer came between us. My body shrank as I starved, and the weight loss was muscle as much as fat. Eventually, I couldn't lift against the weight of the cancer, and because I wasn't lifting, I got even weaker.

Going back to the gym was easy. The gym, after all, is where I was supposed to be, but being there turned out to be very hard. It wasn't just that I was weak; it was that I couldn't exert myself enough to explode in the effort—all I could do was push some tiny weight around and get tired. I could do the work, but I couldn't get the buzz. Then, sometime, maybe this week, maybe last, it turned around. I was completely inside my push on the weights, and that last, muscle-tearing repetition left me flying away, muscles humming at the frequency of myself. It was just like old times.

RADIATION DAYS

No pictures now. I'm still pretty scary to look at, but something has shifted, some quantity has become a quality. The weights are lighter, but the bright, blue glow of that last rep is as heavy as ever. I'm very grateful.

BIGSS and BIHC

∼ BIGSS is Before I Got Sick Syndrome. It's pronounced "bigs." BIHC is Before I Had Cancer and is pronounced just like you want it to be pronounced. They're crutches (one for each arm) for when you have to answer questions about yourself and you think that answers are different Before and After.

It's almost like you have to explain who you are now, or disown it a little. Hey, I may be a spavined, dewlapped, forgetful hawker of odd expectorations, but listen, buddy: I used to be somebody! I was strong, I was handsome, I was smart, I gulped red wine and sipped red lips. There was life here. Understand? (OK, so I lied about the handsome part.)

Well, no, they don't understand, and they shouldn't, but who can blame you for trying? Sometimes you know who you were better than who you are now, sometimes you're sick and bored with confronting your new reality, and sometimes it's just too damn sad.

And the only power you have over the situation is getting over it. Right. Accept it and amazing things start to happen. If you can't really accept it, at least find it funny. Maybe it will go away; maybe you will. Either way, it's just temporary, and, frankly, it always was.

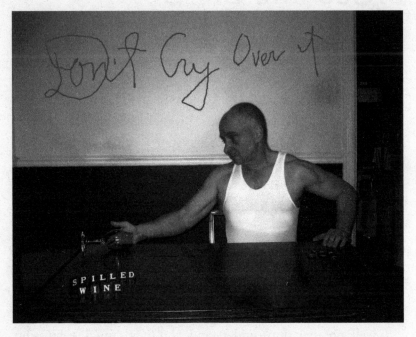

It's a BIHC: if you spilled the claret, little brother, mop it up and find another.

It's Not Like That Anymore

～ Here's what I remember about the ball game: there was a moment when everything went quiet. Number 42 on third base, looking runner-ish; you could hear a guy clear his throat from three sections away. Full count, two on, two out; everybody inhaled and held it. Robinson scored; Brooklyn won.

Last night at the Phillies-Brewers game, there wasn't a moment of quiet, more like a constant roar, a jet engine with bad taste in music.

Here's another thing: a ticket used to be cheap; last night's was sixty bucks. So it used to be that you could go to the game anytime, any impulse. See every team in the league at least once? Sure. Leave a boring game or a rainy one and catch the ninth at your local? Why not? These days, you've got an investment in the damn thing.

But nothing's like it used to be, and it's still the ballgame, and it's still great. I never told you this before, but one of my thoughts when the surgeon told me that most folks in my situation die was that I was not going to see this baseball season. Too bad—the locals have the best pitching they ever had, probably the best in the league. Now, I can hear you saying that pitching alone never got anybody to the World Series, but so what? A beautiful season is something to be grateful for, like that one night at the Eastman Institute with that Nureyev guy on stage or the sweet corn from a field south of Fulton, New York. Like that.

151

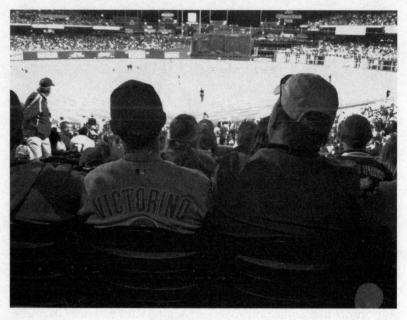

Bottom of the twelfth.

So, when my friend Jim Shrader called and invited me to the game, it was a chance to peek in on a show that I never thought I'd get to see. (Jim knew all that, but he's not the kind of guy to talk about it, just mentioned a ball game and a beer; would I mind coming out on a cool spring night?)

The omens started out bad. Lots of Pilsner at the concession stands, some Pale Ale, none of the really good local stuff. Our starting pitcher was the number five starter. We settled for Guinness cans. We settled for the starter. Then the misplays started. Our shortstop looked like he was hungover, and grounders through the middle were automatic base hits. There were errors, five of them. We took the lead; they tied. We went to two to one; they tied again. Extra innings, top of the twelfth, they score three, we don't, it's over.

It's Not Like That Anymore

But there's another view of things. Guinness in the can isn't all that bad. The moon was full (full moon over the ball park—can you see it?) and the weather was perfect; the tension was great (extra innings!). The seats were just to the first base side of home, so we had as good a view of the pitchers as the batters did—I hope the guy who did my root canal had seats like these. The guy in front of us was wearing a Victorino jersey. Phillies fans will recognize the name of one of our outfielders, but I think that *Victorino* obviously means "little victory." Little victory? Damn right it was.

Thanks, Jim. Any time you want, just take me out to the ball game.

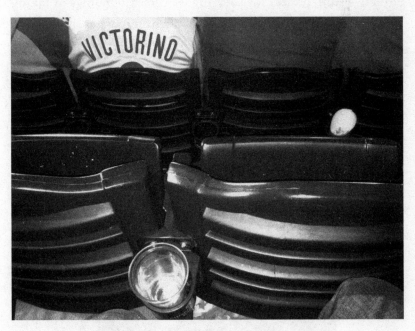

Little victory, folded chair, stadium beer cup.

Wood Violets

꙳ When I first started walking in Carpenter's Woods, the ground near the Heyward Street entrance was covered with English ivy. It's attractive stuff, perfect for covering university buildings or taking the place of a lawn. Unfortunately, this alien creeper has spread from gardens to forest, and it's done a lot of damage.

It not only choked out all the native plants that the bugs and the birds need to live, but it climbed the trees, eventually killing them by smothering the leaves or by making them so top-heavy that they broke. It was pretty dispiriting to watch the stuff spread deeper and deeper into my woods, knowing that in ten or twenty years or so, there would be no native forest floor.

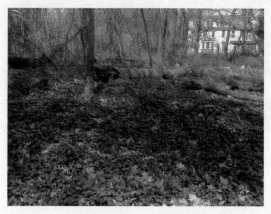

Even the fallen leaves don't stop English ivy.

Wood Violets

What made it worse was that another beautiful invader, Norway maple, was crowding and shading out our native trees. We were headed for a forest that was totally lovely, completely green, and thoroughly sterile.

Since none of our native bugs and worms lives on and around the new species, it wouldn't be long before the birds that live off of them would stop visiting. We're losing wildlife habitat to development all the time; how much more bitter to have forest that looks like habitat but isn't.

Then, about three years ago, somebody started to pull the stuff up. Every time there was a heavy rain or a melt after a snowstorm, I'd see piles of stringy little ivy corpses piled up just off the paths in the woods. This public-service gardener picked one area to make ivy-free and steadily expanded it. I used to smile at the earnest naiveté of the person who thought her hands would make a difference against this green bio-tsunami, but it was nice that someone took arms against a sea of tendrils.

But two years ago in spring, the cowslips came back where the ivy had been. A few young trees, poplars and cherry mostly, started to pop up. That summer there were butterflies—the Azures that lived on the cherries—and then we saw robins scrounging for worms.

This week, after a long, rainy spring, there were wood violets just inside the entrance. Wood violets!

There's one patch in the photo, but there were dozens more and lots of individual plants scattered where the ivy had been. A person could get sloppy with the metaphors, and we have enough allegories available to make Dante sigh, but that would be too easy. It's shirtsleeve weather, there are deep purple flowers underfoot, and, for the moment at least, we have won.

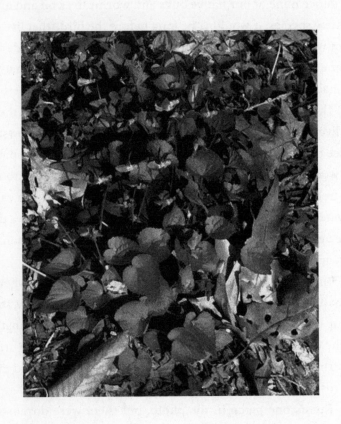

No Longer Handicapped, Symptoms Return

～ It's time to put away the handicapped placard that gives the sick special parking privileges. Not that I don't love special privileges, but a wise person told me once that if you pretend to a disastrous hurt, the universe will make an honest man out of you. The truth is that right now, I'm strong enough to walk, thank you. So just to avoid the yucky karma, it's time to put the blue plastic gimme card away and circle the block like everybody else. Shit.

For the last week or three, I've been having a return of the symptom that started this whole thing: a stabbing pain in my right ear canal. It just happens from time to time, maybe twice or three times a day now. It lasts only for a few seconds, and in the context of life lately, it ain't much. But it's omen-ous, so I'll get it checked out at Fox Chase. In the meantime, it's still spring, and it's nice to have that blue thing out of my car.

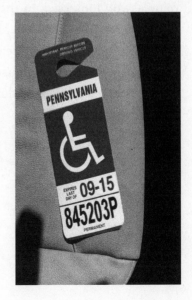

Life Summary: Regrets

～ Every quote I could find about regret involves somebody bragging about how they don't traffic with regrets, how they put that stuff behind them and got on with whatever was getting on. I like the idea of living regret-free, and I don't have much in my own active regret account. There's no doubt that people can make little godlets out of their regrets, even use them to explain themselves out of doing something in the here and now. So, hooray for the jazz singer snapping out "No Regrets."

But something's missing in all this existentialist bravado: there's value as you look back in the things you did badly, in the times you were less when more was called for. I'm not recommending hair shirts or anything penitential, more like an honest embrace, a self-forgiveness without excuses. I can't say that I have the map for this particular Middle Path down yet, but, being in a summarizing mood, here's where I am.

regrets in april

last fall you dropped regrets along the forest floor
the fresh ones just remembered
the ones you aged in casks
of explanation oak
the ones you kept and
the wons you lost.

Life Summary: Regrets

the ones you grew out of and
the ones that grew out of you
and maybe the bhikku who takes care of you
(the buddha ranger pointing out danger)
trailed along behind and carrying a few regrets that
were just out of your reach,
tossed them farther off the trail until
like yellow leaves in the opal-gray light of autumn dawn
there was a regret-filled frosting and then forgetful winter.

it's april now. (you will not die 'til late, late summer)
and along the dirt-scented trail
regret's seedlings are arrayed,
forgiving, laughing, filled with beer and whistles
and in the woods the sprouts of the only all
you could be are bending slightly spritely with the
birdish burden of a new generation
singing, calling like to like,
fortifying, leathering their nests,
forgiving last autumn's leaves
and dancing, calling in the light.

Tombstoning

Tombstoning, verb: To accumulate accolades or accomplishments whose main purpose is to further your career after you're dead.

I just found out that I'm going to be awarded an honorary degree. Now, you probably know somebody with an honorary degree—a doctorate, maybe, or an LLD, but I'll bet I'm the first person you know who's got an honorary associate's degree and who's this happy about it. Here's the story:

Once upon a time, I started a culinary arts program at a local university. Back then, the idea of somebody studying culinary arts—learning to cook, learning to nourish—was just outlandish. College folks thought chefs were like car mechanics, people who trained somewhere else, took care of their occasional needs, and definitely didn't wear mortarboards or attend faculty meetings. So, there was a lot of resistance in college circles, and if it weren't for the president liking the idea, it never would have happened: we ended up offering the first bachelor's in culinary arts in the country. It was a step toward chefs being seen as professionals, and while it doesn't compare to what the Food Network did, it helped change the way people thought about the people who cook for them.

One of the odd resistances that I met was from people in the university who asked me where I got my culinary degree. I don't have one. In fact, the option didn't exist for me back in the old days, and I was making the whole thing up from scratch. But academics being what academics are, they always got to raise an eyebrow, and everything I had to say about the importance, the seriousness, and the beauty of cooking was diminished.

All this was a long time ago, and there are culinary degrees all over the country now. Better yet, people who love to cook can entertain the idea that they have a calling, a craft, a profession, and that it's at least as serious as, let's say, cost accounting or clothing design or turf management or any of dozens of other things that you can study in college.

I love this stuff; I take it seriously. Even more so, I love the kids who love this stuff. I rejoice in the chances they have that food nerds in my generation didn't. I'm glad that the gender crap is gone, and I'm glad there's an audience for careful work and a career ahead for careful workers. It looks like my teaching days are over, and what happened to me doesn't matter so much now. But.

The Academy of Culinary Arts is granting me an honorary degree in culinary arts. It's an associate's degree. It's the degree that people get after two years of showing up for six-hour classes at odd times of the day, after working a job or two and then dragging themselves to school and hoping that their kids and their spouses don't hold it against them. It's a hardscrabble degree; it smells like fry-max, and it looks like a pile of soup bones, and I'm so happy that I might cry.

To celebrate, J and I went out to dinner at Fuji. (When somebody says they're taking me out and I can pick the place, it's usually Fuji.) We didn't order; we just nodded to the chef, and the food started coming, and one—monkfish liver and caviar in a citrus broth—looked like this:

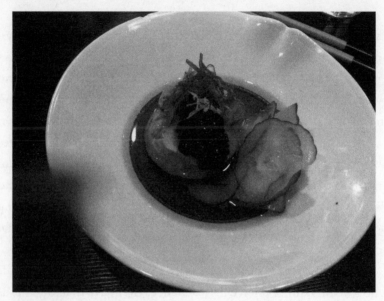

and another one looked like this:

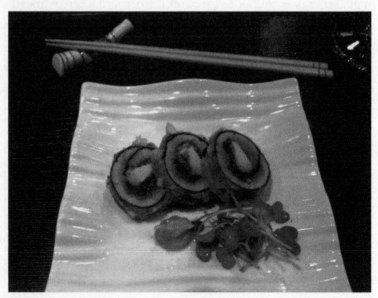

I think there may be something to this culinary stuff, and now I've got the degree to prove it.

Here's What Matters

～ I've been hoping that somehow this cancer would lead me to a few big ideas. I sort of have the idea that the whole business would be worthwhile if I came out of it—or at least came to the end of it—a little bit smarter than when I started. I haven't been completely disappointed, as you know if you've been reading this and managed not to gag at any of my matched pearl-handled epiphanies.

Today's new big idea started with a weird telephone call. It was from the manager in a Center City restaurant—a Japanese place where I've never been. The nice young man wanted me to know that a certain Jeffrey Smith had called him and wanted to buy me dinner, and asked when I would like to come in.

Jeff was a student of mine back in the Nixon years. He was an army veteran, doing college on a Vietnam scholarship. I was a graduate student teaching something or other. We talked a lot, and after he left school, we caught up with each other every decade or so—bars in New York, cantinas in Miami. No small talk—there never was time—just the rush of "Whataya know?" and "Ain't it great?"

Anyway—I was deeply moved by his gesture; I might have been a little weepy even. It wasn't the dinner; it was the sheer kindly genius (generosity plus originality) of the thing, and it brought back all the flames of kindness that have come my way since this damn thing started. The rides to radiation and the bowls of soup and visits and the smiles pointing to the right direction when I thoroughly lost my way. In fact, when I thought about all those acts, all that generosity—when I herded all those little lights together—the effect was blinding. I was dazzled into thinking that maybe kindness is the only thing that matters. Not wit, not accomplishment, not even getting your poems published or seeing your kid do OK in law school. Yeah, maybe kindness is the big human Everest. How the hell did I miss that all these years?

I called Jeff to thank him, and he told me—in a rush of his own poetry—what was behind his picking up the tab for dinner for the cancerman: he was thinking about some things I said to him, some things that he thought were helpful, some things that he thought were kind. Not necessarily clever or beautiful, but kind. Big wheel keeps on turnin', don't it?

I probably should have known this—Manny Hoffman was kind and generous to most people, Mary Grace Hoffman—when she wasn't racked by fear—was, too. I've always been attracted to kindly people: my ex-wife, her mom, J, Gilmore, Brigitte, Peter, the friends that mean the most to me (you know who you are). I even had two great dogs as teachers, but, alas, I've always been a little too defensive to be truly kind—in spite of all those good examples.

It took throat cancer and a dinner tab to make the point: so, ladies and gentlemen, I'd like to propose a toast:

To Kindness and the Kindly; no art and no artist are closer to the Divine, more soaked in the Buddha-nature, more noisily beautiful, more quietly grand.

How to Beat Cancer

∼ I went to a meeting of the Wissahickon Brewers' Guild the other night. There was serious beer tasting, some serious talk about the difficulties of grinding unmalted wheat berries, some homemade cheese, a dozen different kinds of beer. Nice folks, very dear, lots of people glad to see me looking less corpse-like. It's a really sweet place to be, and that's not even counting the beer. Somebody said, "So, you beat cancer? Congratulations. How did you do it?"

The main truth of the matter, the first thing, is this: you don't beat cancer; it beats the shit out of you, steals a year, takes your taste buds, your voice, and any damn thing else. And that's if you're lucky. You may live through it, buddy-buddy, but you sure don't beat it.

There are actually only two ways to beat cancer, and, again, with luck, you can do 'em both. The first one is dying from something else first. Fire your cardiologist, take up skydiving, or move to a really bad neighborhood. Naa-nanny-boo-boo, cancer!

The best one is this: if you live until spring, you take your dog for a walk in the woods. Maybe there's a tree in flower; maybe the dog sits under it. Maybe she turns slightly blue and becomes the other blue dogs in your life. Maybe she sits there under the tree looking like she'd fix it for you if she could, but she'll wait for you at the end either way. Maybe all your dogs rush out from the stream behind the tree and nuzzle your hand. The day that happens, you beat cancer.

RADIATION DAYS

. . .

Earaches are getting worse. The dentist tells me that the little lump I'm feeling in my mouth is an oral papilloma, and she doesn't want to do any work on my teeth until after the oncologist looks at it. She added something about zapping it with a laser. I don't imagine they'll let me drive the laser myself, but I'll let you know exactly how much fun the zapping is.

The Health Benefits of Cancer

∿ I saw my cardiologist, Irv Herling, this week. He's a serious physician and a good guy. I haven't been in his office in a year and a half, so the last time he saw me, I weighed about fifty pounds more than I do now. When he sees me, he does a really good job of looking like he's not looking shocked. Mostly he's empathizing—he examines the tattoos that they used to focus the radiation; he notes the lump where the chemo port is. He's a bit of a Yiddishist, so as he clucked, I said, "For this, you kept me alive?" but his long face made me regret it immediately.

Then, gradually, we go over my lab report. If I had studied up for the blood test, I couldn't have done better. My cholesterol is lower than my IQ (which itself is declining fast). The good cholesterol and the bad cholesterol are identical. If my triglycerides were expressed in $1,000 bills, you couldn't buy a Lexus. Glucose? He notes that it's a bit low.

All this good news is driven by weight loss. Skinny people have healthier hearts, they say. I've been thinking about a self-help health book. Title ideas include *Benign Malignancies*, *The X-Ray Diet*, and, for the beauty market, *Be a Chemo Dreamboat*.

Have a Nice Day
(if You Dare)

∼ Today, I drove through the Pine Barrens to a little meadow near the Atlantic Culinary Academy, and, with gray clouds rolling by overhead, sat through a pretty decent commencement speech and walked away with my culinary arts degree. Now, there are more layers in that experience than in a well-made croissant, and during the long drone of calling the graduates, I got to think about most of them. Sweet. Bitter. The whole complicated business of sweet, delayed recognition and the sense, as the young people filed up one by one by never-ending one, of time passing by was like a morality play. I think the moral was something like "The Impermanence of Things." Or maybe it was "Use More Salt and Drink Better Wine." Hard to tell.

Anyway, I spent an hour after the ceremony hanging out with the faculty, watching them pack up and head off for summers as personal chefs or culinary tour guides. These are remarkable, focused people, extraordinarily dedicated to their profession and their students. Good guys. The dean, Kelly McClay, is a mensch, or maybe that should be a menschette. They mostly seem to like me; I certainly liked being with them. If you've ever had a gang at work—people who made you glad you punched in—you know what I mean.

Then I came home, and in the mail, there was a magazine called *Off the Coast* (Spring 2011). No, it's not about littoral assassination;

it's one of those literary jobs, and I had a poem in it. The poem is called "The Would-Be Lepidopterist," and I think I already told you about it. It's about a fellow who never really made anything of himself because he spent too much time admiring the bugs and smelling the flowers. It's about missed opportunities and the penalty you pay for a lack of steely, business-like focus. There's this bit:

> *No eternity for those bugs or you*
> *Just a messy, scaly insect stew*
> *No dry forever on a pin*
> *Just vanished scale on a dusty wing.*

The poem actually verges close to the edge of expressing regret, but it's saved at the end by a towel-snap of irony.

Happy hit number three for the day. In fact, I was on a happy roll. Yesterday and the day before, I spent time with my daughter. Sweet time, rare time, and you know how pathetic we overinvolved parents can be about stuff like that.

So, how did I feel? All that good feeling left me feeling suddenly scared—worried about my trip to the surgeon tomorrow, as if the sweetness of the days gave me more to lose. Maybe for the first time, I felt vulnerable.

And then Olghods (Our Lady of Getting Hip to your Own Dumb Self) paid me a visit while I was drinking a farmhouse ale and thinking things over. "The good stuff," she whispered, "has to be endured, too." Then she nibbled my earlobe. "Be brave," she said. "It's a lot less work."

The Good Surgeon and the Good News

❧ The surgeon says, "Don't bite me!" as he gets ready to make you want to do just that. His voice is angry, urgent: "Don't bite me, or else I'll run this ocean liner up on the damn iceberg, y'hear?" he seems to be saying.

Then it's the old shoehorn in the mouth, fist down the throat, hot sterilized mirror on your cheeks and tongue.

He's gonna do a biopsy of the little growth. Probably a harmless papilloma, he says, but we gotta make sure. He also schedules another PET scan for the end of June. This is the so-called "gold standard" of cancer detection in the head and neck, but as I remember, we went off the gold standard a few decades back and for good reason. The exam is over in five minutes, my insurance company is billed, and I'm walking to the garage by myself feeling slightly bored.

Burnholme Park surrounds the Fox Chase Cancer Center campus, and the trees are in full summer leaf. It's cool and damp, and I drive away glad that I lived to see it and glad that I can think of this visit as just part of a dull routine.

• • •

We have dinner at the brewpub with the Gilmores, spend a couple of hours with Oscar Wilde at the theater across the street, and head to J's house full of beer and contentment. There's an email waiting for me. I quote:

The Good Surgeon and the Good News

Hi Lynn,

We're interested in your beer book—how would you feel about doing it in color? Either you could provide the images or we could give you access to our stock photos sites and you could find the pertinent images.

Let me know if that's something that interests you and we can discuss details!

Best,

Jenn

I'm too sleepy to react much; all I feel is happy and proud. Another one of my babies is gonna do all right, with me or without. It's a three-book year, and so to bed.

Don't Starve!

∼ This chapter is for you readers with your own cancer drama. Everybody else, skip to the bottom of the chapter where there's a wry little ditty about food and cooking.

· · ·

Are they gone? Good.

Why should I be the only one who gets some good ideas from this cancer-go-round of mine? I discovered a solution to a problem that may come up for you. I pretty much stopped eating around the end of my radiation. I couldn't swallow very well, my mouth was too dry for me to chew properly, and I was nauseated most of the time. I got no help from a bunch of anti-nausea drugs, and there's no medical marijuana in Pennsylvania. I kept track of my intake for a while: seven hundred calories a day on the average, maybe one thousand on a good day.

So, naturally, the weight melted off me. How much? It's hard to know where to start counting, but maybe I was 175 pounds (80 kilograms) when this started and 133 pounds (60 kilograms) at the worst. I may have already mentioned that I looked like a Peking duck without the shellac or one of those guys from the Bataan death march. By a body-fat calculation that I had done about a year before the diagnosis, I had 153 pounds (70 kilograms) of lean body mass.

Don't Starve!

That means that I was losing muscle, maybe ten kilos of it. Wasting away, "Streets of Philadelphia" and all that.

But enough about me. Here's what I wish I had known. Forget about tricking yourself into eating. Nothing's going to taste good, and you're not going to be hungry. What you need is something that acts like food and goes in like medicine. Something you can decide to swallow that will preserve your muscle and won't make you vomit.

Here's what I want you to do—it worked for me after the worst of the nausea had gone. Assemble the following:

Whole-grain, high-protein cereal, like Kashi Go Lean
Protein powder
Fruit, fresh or frozen
Definitely a ripe banana
Milk, and maybe some yogurt

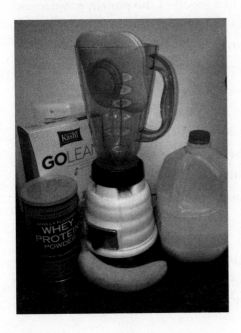

Remember the banana: just think of William Tell shooting one off his kid's head.

RADIATION DAYS

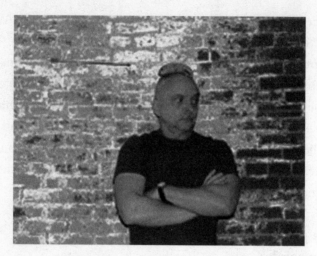

William Tell, looking out for arrows.

Measure a cup (250 milliliters) of the cereal into a blender jar. Add the fruit and a cup or more of milk. Blend it thoroughly until the mixture loses its grit. Add a scoop of the protein powder and blend some more. If you use frozen fruit, the result will be thick and cold and easily worth 450 calories and thirty grams of protein. The whole-grain cereal is also high in fiber, which takes care of that other digestive problem that we don't talk about much.

Stock up on frozen berries and mangoes if you can; use flavorings if they help you (I made vanilla extract from a Madagascar vanilla bean and grain alcohol). Whey protein is absorbed quickly; casein protein leaves you feeling full—take your pick. Make a breakfast date with yourself every morning and slam one of those down. I never tried adding a shot of rum, but why not? What harm can it do? Give you cancer?

Focus on breakfast. In the morning you'll feel as close to hungry as you ever will. For the rest of the day have one of those liquid meal substitutes handy and cold. I used one called Ensure. How does it taste? I don't know. I could smell the cocoa in the "chocolate" one; the vanilla was just cold and smooth and soothing. It was also pretty good medicine for dry mouth.

Oh. One other thing:

for r.y.[‡‡]

imagine this: you hear:
"oh, you remember x?" him, oh yeah.
"he's sick" and then imagine that you start thinking
about x and so you google him, call him and you talk and
x tells you that if the tumor don't get him, the cure sure will.
and imagine you knew that a thoroughly illegal marijuana ganache
would improve his outcome (as they say) no matter what the outcome be
and imagine that you just decide that you're going to send
this old cornerboy what he needs just what he needs now.
and, not being crazy, you know that there's a risk
and you decide to mother-fuckin' do it anyway.
well then you just imagined yourself
a being to be.
imagine that.

I'm back at the gym now, and I weigh just under 150 pounds, and I still have my morning shake. If this helps, let me know. If you have other ideas about fooling the appetite and saving the body, let me know, and I'll pass them on. Most important thing: don't starve.

• • •

[‡‡] It's too bad that I can't tell you who r.y. is, or if he or she is even a real person who took a risk to send me some magic medicine when I was starving to death. Everybody needs an r.y. now and again.

RADIATION DAYS

Kitchen Philosophies

The old chef said, "At the end of the day,
how you practice is how you play."
The pastry chef had a different view:
"Don't waste your truffles and cutlets on stew."
The apprentice listened and couldn't agree
she said, "the best thing out of this kitchen is me."
(Bennie the fry cook just sat on his ass
and drank red wine from a water glass.)
Ramon, the dishwasher, ventured a joke
as he took a break for a nip and a smoke.
"It's a very good day when I give it my best
and don't hear a word from the INS.
Say what you'll do and do what you say—
the rest is all compost and gets carted away."

A Dinner Party

 J and I had dinner last night with Hugh and Janet Gilmore. Nothing effortful, just an end-of-the-week, shared takeout nosh. We sat on the deck in their backyard eating Thai food and drinking beer and listening to the catbirds calling out for love and a one-bedroom condo in Chestnut Hill.

These are the kind of friends who let you drop the barriers a bit, and we came to the part of the evening—the mango and sweet rice dessert—when you tell the truths about your families. Hugh asked me something about my parents—he wondered if my mother's Irish family thought she was going to hell for marrying a Jew. I had to tell him that it was both worse and better than that. Worse because she became Jewish herself (a Jewess, they used to say) and better because my mom's sisters loved my father. They doted on him in a way that's almost impossible to imagine these days. They even called him—their brother-in-law—"Uncle Manny." One aunt always brought him a footstool when he sat in her living room; another would fetch the ashtray.

I guess they indulged him partly because he was an unashamedly doting husband, and partly because he was generous with them in a way that they had heard about but never experienced. He did so much right by them that they thought he could do no wrong.

RADIATION DAYS

Anyway, somehow in the middle of telling this story, I started to cry. It's not a sad story, except in the way that all our stories are sad, but I had pointed a dousing rod at some big spring of sadness, and I kept on with my story, crying into some very good beer (Victory Golden Monkey in the big bottle).

So, later, I found myself wondering where that rush of lugubriousness came from. I'm not especially sentimental about my father: he and I did the best we could, but we managed only moments of closeness. No blame, just different souls. As I tried to puzzle it out, it seemed to me that I wasn't remembering him so much as I was living for a minute in his time, sensing his loneliness, maybe rolling it up into mine. Maybe we just naturally travel back in time as we get older. Or maybe it's just time to say how much I miss what I missed and time to give it the crying that it's due. I guess it could be that I'm sad that I'm finishing up without having earned that sort of love, or maybe it just reminded me that my kid and I may be no closer than Manny and his kid.

It was a good, unstoppable cry, one that may have even washed away the regret that set it off. Our hosts didn't look too embarrassed, and we all pay the meat bill eventually—so why not throw in a little salt?

The Examined Head, or Dr. Galloway and the Snot Scope

～ Did you ever wonder how they check out a cancer on the back of your tongue?

Yesterday, I was back at Fox Chase seeing Tom Galloway. He's the radiation specialist. He's also the doctor who takes time to answer my questions. Of course, the thing he wants to know the most is if all his radiation killed the cancer or not. I've had two biopsies since November; neither of them were conclusive. We'll also be repeating the PET scan in a couple of weeks; the last one was also—you guessed it—inconclusive.

So, Dr. Galloway wants to take a look. Most people gag when they're touched around the back of the tongue, so any peeking has to be sort of indirect. Here's what they do: they snake a long rubber hose up through your nostril and around and down your throat. It's an evil-looking thing, and we may well call it the snot scope. There's a light and a lens on the end of the hose, and it's connected to an eyepiece in the examiner's hand.

I wouldn't call it painful, but there's a definite creepy sense of invasion. Every muscle in your body seems to be tensed and ready to get you and your poor head out of that chair and away from that thing. "Creepy" is an odd, compound feeling. As near as I can tell, creepy is made up of *fear* and *disgust*. Think of a miniature version of a colonoscopy—without the redeeming anesthetic before and fresh-squeezed orange juice immediately after. Think of something that might properly be done to a suspected terrorist who's swallowed his cell phone or a dog who ate your engagement ring.

I can tell you that one doesn't get used to the snot scope—at least this one doesn't. I'm surprised they don't need a surgeon to excise my back from the examining chair when the procedure is over. However, I was reminded of something useful. Galloway had a resident insert the scope and peer around before the eyepiece was handed over to him. This increased my up-your-nose-with-a-rubber-hose time by about 120 percent, and my discomfort by about double that.

What I want to pass on is this useful realization: even when there are sound educational motives and worthy humane values involved, it's OK to tell the doctor that you'd rather not be examined by the trainees. (If they put that thing in you and then went out for beer and kielbasa, you'd object, wouldn't you?) "Please, good sir or madam, just creep me out yourself and do it as efficiently as possible."

I don't want to suggest that you should refuse every student examination. We do have some obligation to our fellow creatures to help train the docs. I'm saying that everybody should feel comfortable saying when they're uncomfortable and that we're all entitled to opt out of one instance of being cadavers before our real cadaverosity.

And Don't Thirst, Either

〜 J reminds me that I was admitted to the hospital twice during my treatment. Both times I was dehydrated. Since this was the dead of winter, I guess you could say I was freeze-dried. The first time I woke up in the middle of the day, walked to the bathroom, and passed out on the way. The second time, I tried to get out of bed, and I folded like overcooked pasta. When J drove me up to the emergency room, I collapsed getting out of the car. Fortunately, the young man who picked me up didn't have to strain much, since I weighed about as much as a standard poodle.

You can ask your Wikidoctor about dehydration, but it's really pretty easy to understand: your body does its work in its own water. Let the water level get too low, and instead of work you get job actions, work stoppages, and industrial protests. Ever had a hangover? Acute dehydration is like that, but worse, and without the preceding exaltation, laughing, shameless flirting, and tearful recitations of Dylan Thomas.

I'm going to save you a lot of research here. The best cure for dehydration is to drink lots of water. It's almost impossible to overdo it—just drink. Then how do we cancer buffs let ourselves get dehydrated if the cure is so simple? Those of us over in the head-and-neck division often find it hard, even painful, to swallow. So we slow our drinking down. If you're over fifty, your thirst response is probably impaired, so you don't drink reflexively any more. And

181

you're nauseated—which makes the thought of swallowing anything unthinkable.

There's a spiral here, a malicious, downward, dizzying slide. The drier you get, the less you want to drink—and the more brittle and unresponsive you become. So you desiccate some more and feel worse and become less capable and even drier.

So, what to do? Conspire against yourself on your own behalf. You're not thirsty, so attach drinking to things you'd do anyway. Make it a point of religion to drink a glass of water or milk or juice every time you wake up. Pay attention to your dry mouth, and treat it with sips of water from the bottle that's now your constant companion. If you speak in public, have a bottle of water with you and use it as a punctuation mark. Consider broth. Praise yourself and drink every time you get up to piss, and learn to love pale urine and be alarmed at the dark variety.

If you're reading this because you love someone who's whirling around in the cancersphere, your new way of saying "I love you" is to offer, then insist on, having a drink together.

Finally, if you have an installed catheter going right into a vein, ask your doctor about taking fluids intravenously. If you're in reasonable condition, you can take a liter of saline in about thirty minutes. You can learn to hook yourself up, get hydrated, and disconnect in the course of about two innings of a typical Phillies game—well, maybe three innings considering the 2011 pitching staff—but you get the idea.

Whatever you do, it's your job to not dry out. Life is wet work. Stay alive; stay damp.

Tripping

Part One

∼ Cancer likes to stay close to home. You can imagine all the reasons: low energy, incredibly fussy diet, outbursts of sentimental attachment to dogs and cats and things and people at home. So one of the signs of a remission, of the time in between scans, is the desire to take a little trip. I wanted to see my friend Peter, and he lives four hours away in place called State College, Pennsylvania, or Happy Valley or Nittany Hill or something. I wanted to see him for a lot of reasons, but the most shallow one is that we laugh a lot together. The most elevated one is that we like a lot of the same things, and if I decide I want to stand by the side of a lake watching little bass cruise the shallows, there's a good chance that he knows just the spot. Sometimes driving is fun, but humping your car down the road is a pretty low-skill, high-alertness job—the sort of thing that tires a person out without the redeeming sense of accomplishing something worthwhile. So I came here by bus. It's about a five-hour run with a change in Harrisburg, but the view is seductive, and since I'm not driving, I get to enjoy it. I drift between my Inspector Montalbano mystery, the beautiful countryside, and the bus-seat version of napping. For the last two hours, my bus had Wi-Fi; it drives up along the Susquehanna, then the Juniata, and everything is green and alive. We've been out to the acre that Peter's restaurant keeps in produce, we've had chicken and beer in the backyard with the Chipping Sparrows, the Blue Jay, and the Cardinals. We've been to the achingly gorgeous front lawn at the Clearwater Conservancy with its butterfat milkweeds and to the luxurious arboretum at Penn State. Peter is one of the few people who understands my obsession with food markets, and, even though he may not share it, he's happy to indulge me with a stroll around Wegman's and an unhurried quarter-hour in their beer department.

Today we kayaked up in Black Moshannon. It's a bog whose black, reflective water is dotted with water lilies and overseen by damselflies. About a mile and a half from our put-in, just past the spot where the Canada Geese and their goslings were working the weeds, we both stopped paddling. We bobbed there for a half hour or so in the broad view of the lilies and the hills and the black-to-blue sky. We watched the little boy in his mud boots bring his treasures to his blonde mommy; we scoot toward land when it looks like thunderclouds. Then Peter says, in a voice that he's obviously borrowed from some indoor person, "Don't you ever get bored just looking at a lake?" It pierces the perfect contentment of the moment in the best way, turns the page without smearing the ink. We laugh, dip paddles, and a half hour later, we're eating sushi and I'm ready for an afternoon nap.

• • •

It's my first kayaking since last fall when I launched my wooden kayak and the next week gave myself up to the treatment. Today, I didn't know if I'd be strong enough, if I could still paddle. It was fine, just fine, and I promise myself to be back on the water again in a few days.

Tripping

Part Two

Sometime last winter, I was recovering from treatment and still unsure if treatment had worked. I was at that two-roads-diverged-in-a-yellow-cancer-clinic moment: uncertain if this cancer was going to get me, but definitely feeling just a little bit better, a tiny bit stronger, and more willing to do things in the world. The first things I did, now that I look back on them, were things that I fancy I'm good at. I wrote poetry, poked out a little fiction. I started to cook again, and I even gave a beer tasting at a time when I didn't even have two taste buds to rub together.

Back from my trip to the woods and friendship, I feel more than a little stronger. I feel like it's time to do something I'm not very good at and have a few laughs as I stumble through it. One of the areas where I'm not quite adequately competent is building stuff. I didn't grow up around mechanics and handy people. My dad and I took each other apart from time to time, but we never disassembled a car engine. Somehow, making and building things just never came up in our two-bedroom apartment in Brooklyn.

But one day in my early thirties, I bought a house. It was, like me, a fixer-upper with real potential. I didn't have much money, so I applied my absolute lack of knowledge and skill to everything that needed doing. I'd love to tell you that hard work and determination triumphed, but in fact the renovation was a series of small flops, big screw-ups, and misplaced ambition, punctuated by occasional successes.

I learned stuff. I never got good at any of it, but I became tolerably "handy." The odd thing is that I also started to like building things. I read the Garrett Wade wish book when my friends were reading the Victoria's Secret catalog. I bought tools; I coveted table saws and routers. I never got good at it, and I never stopped.

My wife, to her great credit, indulged me, and occasionally I overachieved and felt really good about it.

So. With that intermittent reinforcement system in place, I decided it was time to build another kayak—a smaller, lighter boat that I could manhandle onto a car roof. The kit's been sitting in J's garage, and today I sliced it open and got to work.

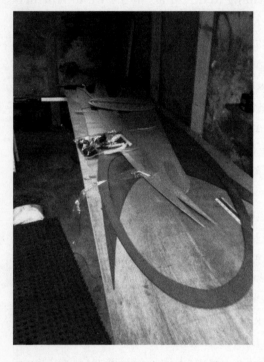

A pile of plywood.

What you see are mostly slabs of four-millimeter plywood that get glued together to make a boat. The first step is to join matching pieces to make bottom, side, and sheer panels. Then you join the two bottom panels to each other, attach the side and sheer panels, throw on a deck,[§§] cover everything in fiberglass, and you got a boat.

___
[§§] Notice the casual "throw on," as if this was all in a day's work for a handy fella like myself.

186

Tripping

Today's work was making the panels by gluing their halves together. To keep up a tradition that I started with my last kayak, I mixed way too much epoxy for the job. That's a total loss, because the stuff sets up like a rock about thirty minutes after it's made. Then I forgot to add a stiffening ingredient to the wet epoxy before applying it. Two good inaugural errors.

Right now the panels are curing overnight, stacked on top of each other and insulated from each other's magic adhesive by sheets of plastic.

How do I feel? Just like old times.

Unrequited Love—Part Two

～ When I was a young man, I was in the Merchant Marine. That means that I was one of the crew who sailed American merchant ships all over the world. I sailed on super-fast cruise ships and cautiously slow freighters. Mostly, I picked ships based on where they were going, and I got some curiosities satisfied.

There was one ship, however, that I lusted to be on. I would not have cared if it went out in the ocean, made a big circle, and came home. I very much wanted to ride *The Big U*.

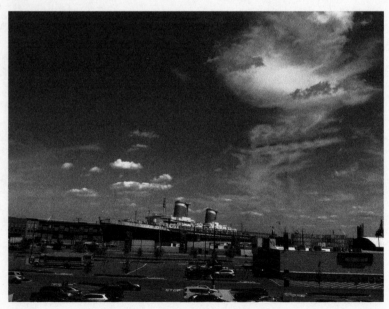

Unrequited Love—Part Two

The Big U was the SS *United States*. It was the fastest thing afloat, and its four screws took it from New York to Southampton (the one in the UK) in three days. Its top speed was gossiped about and rumored to be a government secret. It was said around the union hall that it could be converted overnight into a troop carrier that could move ten thousand soldiers and their equipment ten thousand miles. The four giant shafts that came out of its steam turbine and turned the screws were so massive that they would deform under their own weight if they were ever allowed to stop rotating. I don't remember the rest of the stories, but it doesn't matter—the ship was a legend, and if you sailed on it, you were part of something mythic, something worthy of New York. Sometimes, from the West Side Highway, I'd see her tied up, slow plumes rising out of her stacks and a crew of attendants swarming around the dock, but every time a berth on *The Big U* came up in the union hall, I would throw in my card, and, seniority being what seniority was, I never got the job.

It's years later, and there are a lot of ships that sailed without me, but this particular one—maybe because the process was so impersonal—has a special smoke of nostalgia about it. These days *The Big U* is tied up on Philadelphia's waterfront, across from the Swedish furniture store, rusting quietly in a city with a sense of history. She will never sail again, of course, and her chances of becoming a hospitality industry asset are oxidizing away every day. Eventually, she'll be scrapped or scuttled. Whenever I go down to visit her now, I feel like we found the same home port, and there's some satisfaction in that.

• • •

The Sands of Time, he said,
Are just the grindings off the Rock of Ages,

RADIATION DAYS

The rock's, in turn, a fragment of
The broken World of Hurt.
Without the Hurt, it's obvious,
He continued
That we'd be out of Time
And instead it's clear
That we have Time to spare,

Yes, she said,
And there's Time enough
for grinding here,
And then there's Time to Go.

Today I went in for another PET scan. They're scanning for tumors, which is sort of like bobbing for apples or trolling for walleyes. The similarity lies in the uncertainty, the wetting your face or tossing your bait and hoping for an apple or a fish.

In this case, we're trying to reduce the uncertainty: Is there a cancerous tumor there or not? Do we have some little malignancy that's set up shop in the thoroughly irradiated and chemically cauterized neighborhood of my throat and planning to go Wal-Mart on me at any moment? Or are we done for a while?

To get ready for a PET scan, I fasted for four hours—no big deal for a guy who didn't eat for weeks. Then Sheldon, witty and kind, poked around in my arm for a while until he found a vein that was willing to accept some radioactive glucose solution. Then I went to a quiet room to rest for a bit while the glucose surged around looking for needy tissue. As I mentioned previously, cancer is especially demanding of glucose, and in a fasting body, it sucks it up faster than the regular muscle tissue. The scan is just a way to eavesdrop on your metabolism (*origliare il metabolismo*)⁵⁵ and see if there are any cells who are just shouting up a storm.

The modern version of the scan has you laying on a table, which slides silently through a big, donut-like machine. The scan takes about twenty minutes, and it's hard not to imagine it as a kind of birth, a sort of passage, or at least a very, very tame ride at a kiddy amusement park.

Today's machine was older, and you slide into an enclosure like a tube sock. I'll give you a dollar if you can do it without thinking the word "coffin." I meditated furiously (yes, that's possible). The technician asked me if I like smooth jazz. No? How about *Classics in Springtime*? Sure. (When you go for your scan, ask to reserve the "open PET scanner" and bring your own iPhone.)

And then it's over, and it's almost noon, and I'm talking to the gorgeous redhead at the coffee bar who tells me that she'd rather be selling red wine, and I'm hungry. I don't think to ask when I'll get the results.

For one thing, Fox Chase has its own rhythm. For another, I'm almost bored with my health; I'd rather think about the boat I'm building or my book bonanza (three books so far this year!) or my next batch of beer or my kid or her boyfriend or anything but me and the reaper.

Truth is, I'm ambivalent about the results. My fantasy is that they say, "You're cancer-free," and I wonder if I'll burnish up or blot out this bright sense of living, of squeezing each day and consciously throwing the rind out the window at night.

Stay tuned.

• • •

---

⁵⁵ Guess who's reading Dante again?

RADIATION DAYS

Today I also saw a pipevine swallowtail butterfly—the first one I've ever seen alive and fluttering. I'll call it a draw.

Yesterday was Father's Day—an American institution that sounds Japanese—I had dinner with my daughter who has become—who'd a thunk it?—a person. Twenty-four years old, poised, thoughtful, humane. A better piece of work than I was at that age, probably better than I am now. I think she is pretty, too, but father eyes are astigmatic that way. Proud? Humbled, actually. In any case, I wanted to applaud. Dinner was good, too.

A Slightly Alloyed Relief

〜 When they refer to the PET scan as the gold standard in cancer diagnosis, they never said anything about pure gold. Nope. The test could be the eighteen-karat standard or even the twelve-, ten-, or eight-. I guess lower karats are possible, too. Maybe the bullion is really bouillon, and what they meant is "the chicken soup standard."

Anyway, I realized that I could be waiting a week or more to find out the results of the scan. I called Tom Galloway's office. (Galloway, you'll remember, is one of those doctors who gives thoughtful, detailed answers to questions.) I told his assistant that I had no problem with bad news over the phone, but I was less comfortable with no news at all, so would they please let me know when the scan had been interpreted?

Dr. Keller called the next day. She is Galloway's apprentice, and I like her, too: for one thing, she seems to be aware that the lump of flesh in the examining chair is a person. For another, *Keller* means cellar, which makes me think of red wine and evocations of lost loves, which are—in this season at least—kind of tender and sweet.

"We have the results of your scan. It showed minimum residual activity of uncertain significance."

"Is the tumor gone?"

"It shows minimum activity."

"Does that mean it's still there and growing?"

"It's of uncertain significance."
"What does that mean?"
"We're happy with the results."

• • •

I ask around. I share my diagnosis with a couple of writers, who understand the language on a deep level, and another doctor who's got a pretty good grasp of how to deliver news. I also give it to someone clerking for a federal judge and who's known for extremely careful and balanced thinking. You might say that I did my own PET scan of the PET scan.

The results are distressingly human: the damn thing is on the ropes. Maybe it's dead; maybe it's just taking a long estival nap. Maybe the radiation killed it; maybe it just pissed it off, and it's plotting revenge. Maybe it will kill you soon; maybe it will kill you later; maybe something else will get you first. Look up "reprieve."

And it turns out that this is just the answer I want. It's very good news, indeed. Yes, the cancer is, for the moment, less of a threat, and, yes, every day I'm alive is a gift. I have some time left, and my best shot is to be ravingly alive for every second of it—to do the things I do well and enjoy the things I do badly, to write and eat and drink and love and travel.

Ah, what's that you say? You got that diagnosis, too? Yup, we all did.

Scheduling Surgery

～ Today it was the oncologist, Barbara Burtness, and her fellow, Pat Boland. Barbara is the one we'll think of as the doctor who managed an education in spite of wasting all that time at medical school. She knows Scandinavian literature, she has opinions about translations of Dante, she raises her eyebrow at my reading him before discussing life and death, and she laughs with relief when I tell her that I keep Epicurus at my bedside.

She has some thoughts for me. The first one is that she sees the PET scan as good news. Cancer, she reminds me, is rarely subtle and never shy. The fact that the active area that lit up the scan is shrinking probably means that the threat is shrinking, too. Hip hip.

And she's concerned about the growth that's sprung up on the floor of my mouth. (Of course mouths have a "floor." They have roofs, don't they?) I've been concerned, too. The new growth is an opportunistic little fellow, expanding like a third-world economy. Let's get it out as soon as possible, OK?

Well, OK. Of course, surgery means a flirt with Death, but Death is our friend, remember? He's the one who reminds us to watch the flight of the flowers and smell the butterflies. So I have to make plans.

The operation itself is a matter of whacking out a piece of lower mouth and seeing what happens to your native song. It reprises, in a way, the questions I had when this whole thing started: Will I be silenced before I'm silenced? If I have to say goodbye to taste, do I have to say goodbye to words? At least this procedure doesn't seem to threaten the taste and smell, although I may have to eat pablum for a while. There may be more radiation or chemo that starts the whole nasty business again, but...No matter, my questions right now are about talk and timing.

My friend Ginni wants to come down from the wilds of upstate Pennsylvania and spend a long lunch. Peter asked me to talk to his students about strategies for selling wine and beer. Dolly wants to scatter the ashes of our old friend McManus. And Julio! Ah, Julio. My old friend is coming in from Vietnam for a day or two. If there were a bodhisattva of charm and education, it would be Julio. (One day Julio ran into my ex-wife. She said, "Knowing you was one of the best things about my marriage." I can't even hold that against him.) A conversation with him is like a night at the opera, Groucho included. A dinner with him is a symposium; lunch is a truly comedic sitcom. For a Spaniard, he's not so bad.

I consult Epicurus. I browse through the Diamond Sutra. The surgery can wait. We'll bake McManus into bread and feed him to the pigeons; I'll lunch with Ginni at the mall. Perhaps my daughter will bring her boyfriend, and we'll have a chat, and Julio and I will condense a year's worth of conversation into a day and a half. Then J and I will go to the ocean, and we'll glide along the bay. I'll indulge my lecture fantasy one last time. There will be oysters and there will be beer, and when I see the good doctor, I'll thank him.

• • •

Today, while I'm getting my blood drawn, there's a throat cancer guy in the chair next to me who looks like I did six months ago. We get to talking, and I find out that he's not eating, and he wonders what I learned. I talk to him about shakes and ganache, and I really wish I could tell him about dancing in the light, or applauding the butterflies, or walking the dog in the woods. But he's got the feeding tube, and everything tastes like ground-up tin cans, and I wish I could cook for him or fool his mouth into taking care of his body. I want to cure him with a frying pan, or at least a blender. The more we talk, the more his face tells me that I can't.

As I leave the bloodsuck room, I realize that all I really hope to gain from this story and this illness is the chance to make it a little better for someone else. It's still all about feeding folks and watching them smile. Why would you recite your own agonies if they didn't lighten the pain of someone else's? I want to stand in front of a room and, instead of telling the people about Italian cooking from 1536 on, let's say, tell them about the humor and power and transformative chill of radiation days.

The Surgeon Takes a Snip

◦ It's biopsy time again.

The doctor is tall and gaunt. He eclipses the hall light when he stands in doorways. He trims his white beard to a stubble, and, even though he heard the message about making small talk with patients, he doesn't really believe it. He barks through his chitchat routine and then goes to the instrument drawer. He's exactly the guy I want right now.

He starts out our meeting with the snot scope. He snakes it up my nostril and down my throat for the eighth or tenth or twentieth time since I've known him. The sense of being invaded by the Housewares and Lawn & Garden section at Lowe's is both undiminished and every bit as pleasant as it always was.

"Say, 'E,' " he says.

"Say, 'Mama.' "

"Say, 'I have no fucking dignity; I'm a series of tubes.' "

OK, maybe he didn't say that last one; maybe he just signed it.

"Don't bite me," he says again as he pushes my tongue around with a shoehorn.

"Breathe through your nose," he tells me as I gag.

The site of the cancer looks pretty good, he says.

We're getting along really well here, and the nurse hands him a syringe with needle. The growth in my mouth, he says, probably

The Surgeon Takes a Snip

hasn't sprouted much in the way of nerves just yet, but this may burn a little. A small pinch is more like it, kind of like finding a piece of shell in the middle of your crab cake. A few seconds later, he's used a little snipper to remove a pinhead's worth of white tissue, and we're done.

"The results will be back in a week," he says. "No, wait. Not a week, I'll be away, twelve days."

"Well, can someone call me?"

Nope.

"I like to look in a patient's eyes when I'm giving them results so that I know they understand the significance of the results."

And what, pray tell, gentle doctor, might the results be? "Is this just a papilloma?"

"That's what we're trying to find out."

"What else could it be?"

"Could be cancer." His eyebrows twitch up a little.

Chemo Brain

～ Some days when I walk Lola in Carpenter's Woods, we meet Jake. He's a yellow Lab whose bounciness is about the same as Lola's. His parent is this lovely creature who might be, if paganism hadn't been eclipsed by the monotheists, a wood sprite. We talk. I mention my kayak building. She says she's never been to the Pine Barrens. I'm shocked. I urge her to go there before the pterodactyls become extinct and the giant turtles shrink to mere dinner-plate size.

Where should she go? Oh, shit. I can't remember the name of the place. It's an outfitter; I rent from them two or three times a year. I give her my email, and by the time she gets in touch, the name comes back to me.

Forgetting Bel Haven Paddle Sports

the name of that kayak rental in the pines
the one where we go all the time,
the one with the cute little whatchamacallit,
yeah, that one.
its name has gone skittering off someplace
into the deeper woods to beat wings with
the date of the battle of mukden and
the name of the girl who taught me how
to eat hardshell crabs with a hammer.

Chemo Brain

in fact, that memory's very being now resembles
that orange butterfly, you know the one
that's named for euclid's something or other?

I know the kayak rental name is right there,
hiding behind the perfect, polished recollection of
all nine cru beaujolais villages
a memory standing in place
with its own nemmo-sign
since, oh, 1975
and the starting lineup of the '55 Dodgers
and the address of Ebinger's bakery
whose last crumb was brushed away thirty years ago.

no matter.
when I go off the trail to find that name,
(murky water paddle daughter shoulda oughter?)
when I go off the trail to find that name,
i'm immune to the poison ivy
and the nits of gnats
and the scratches of lying wineberry.
it only takes two steps, three at the most
and I am in the siren sunshine of the
Bright Indefinite Orchard
picking paunchy fruit from a thousand trees
that I never could have seen
from spots
along the well-remembered, foot-polished trail.

New York Again

~ We're waiting for yet another biopsy report, so it seems only right that we go to New York for a few days. I remind J on the way up about the Titans. No, not the short-lived football team, the legendary giants who were children of a union between the gods and Mother Earth. J, ever obstetrical, wonders about the details of conception and parturition, but I lead her gently back to the metaphorical way of thinking. You see, the Titans gained strength when they touched the earth—their mother—and I've held the suspicion/superstition that New Yorkers do the same. Foot on the ground in one of the five boroughs and an energy surges back into you. Time to go be in places with names like SoHo and Red Hook and Bay Ridge.

The air is warm and the streets are lively. We let ourselves be manipulated by our surroundings. We see the German Expressionist show at MoMA and despair for humanity; we have a beer in a bar on Grand Street and feel like there's hope. I buy a pair of traveler's chopsticks. She looks at shoes. I'm eating these days, able to chew up lots of soft things, so I eat sushi and brioche and slurp down bone marrow and pizza and oxtails and soup dumplings and fried anchovies. J tells me that I'm still painfully skinny. "Bones" she says, as she presses her hand to my chest. For her sake, I have an extra Guinness or two, but I'm so happy to be able to taste and chew and swallow. It's hard to care about *skinny*, I tell her, when back in January, we were thinking about *dead*.

Kaleidoscope

There's a journal called *Kaleidoscope*. No, it's not about looking at mirrored patterns in an altered state of consciousness. It's actually about "Exploring the Experience of Disability through Literature and the Fine Arts." Issue number sixty-three just showed up today, and it has this poem:

Bijou the poodle
—for hs

Bijou the poodle
Pulls Hal the poet
Through the streets
Around the edge
Of Carpenter's Woods.

Poetical Hal has Parkinson's and
Bijou has a lust for bikers and runners
That's not completely wholesome.

Hal can't let Bijou run loose
In the deep of the woods
And Hal is too kind
to keep Bijou inside.

So, lunging at joggers and jerking on leads
Hal and Bijou whirl on,
Leashed together for blocks and blocks
In orbit around the beautiful woods
And each other.

RADIATION DAYS

Because Hal (the poet) and
Bijou (the poodle)
Are both remarkably strong and
Each unwilling to give up
The sweet gyration of
Sliding over the ground
That passes beneath all six of their feet.

(Published in *Kaleidoscope*, 2011)

I wrote this BIHC, and sent it off sometime in the middle of treatment. Today, when I read it in the magazine—a lovely glossy, by the way—I wondered who, exactly, I was writing about. Whoever I was thinking about, I wish man and dog all the best.

You Say, "Hyperplasia,"
I Say, "Po Tah Toe"

～ It took us twelve days to get together to discuss the results, but John Ridge wastes no time on his way into the room. "It's not malignant. It's a hyperplasia." (Incidentally, if you're going to deliver life-or-death sort of news, this is one of the humane ways to do it.) I get it, but how bad is that?

It turns out that on the scale of Good Cells Gone Bad, hyperplasia is still the kid who steals a pack of gum from the candy store. The medical advice? Slap the little bastard before he turns to robbing banks armed with a sub-machine gun and accompanied by a gang of meth-crazed buddies.

Fair enough. How do we do that? Well, it involves General Anesthesia (I knew him when he was a captain). The mouth will be a little messed up afterward, so we schedule the surgery for the end of August, after I get back from Vietnam.

• • •

This visiting professor business is improving. Last season it was New Jersey; next month it's Vietnam. This gig happened because my old boss, Julio, from the end of my teaching career is now the dean of the hospitality management school at Hoa Sen University in Saigon. They needed someone to teach the young hospitality professionals about wine and beer, and I was invited.

RADIATION DAYS

This has all the makings of an adventure. Consider:

- I've never even been on mainland Asia before.
- When I chanted, "Hell no, we won't go," I was talking about this place.
- The food.
- I'll be with an old friend whose company I admire—in a setting where we are both strangers. I'm pretty good at the stranger business, he is a master.
- There will be students with a world view totally different from mine and I'll have the job of explaining my world to them.

I should be trembling with excitement and I'm not. Instead, I'm happy—just happy, filled with a pleasant, warm anticipation. I knew about this last week, and I didn't rush to tell you about it. What's up?

I think the cancer changed me. When I was given the gift of knowing that all that matters is what's happening now, I gave up my fear of dying; I also gave up the wild excitement of anticipation. I'm not there now; maybe I'll be there later, maybe I won't.

In the meantime, there's a dog to walk, and I've got to pack.

Hypermetaphorosis Sets In

~ Walking along the edge of Carpenter's Woods, Lola and I pass by this dead bush honeysuckle. It's been sprayed with herbicide. Now, normally, the victim of hypermetaphorosis sees something like this and makes a leap to images of death by chemistry and gets morbid or at least morose. Next thing you know, *Eunoymus alatus* is spreading like you-know-what, or cancer is curling up the leaves of life; a poisoned summer becomes an early winter, and the sun's warmth goes unheeded, and growth is no more. Yuck.

Don't think I succumbed to that particular illness. Oh, no. I knew that the foresters had been through and sprayed the invasive plants that were reducing the amount of wildlife habitat in the woods. And I knew that this apparent destruction was really just clearing the way for more life, that sometimes what looks healthy, ain't—and that there's more and better life to grow in that spot.

I guess you get where I'm going with this. I'm sorry. I promise to stop soon. Maybe just one or two more in Thailand and another itty-bitty metaphor in Vietnam. Then I'll quit. Really.

• • •

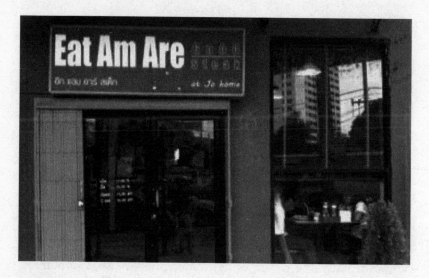

Could you have said it better yourself? In this English-as-ideogram restaurant sign in Bangkok, you've got the whole post-cancer proposition nicely stated. If I eat, I am, and, by the way, if we eat together, we are. I think of Hugh Gilmore's column The Enemies of Reading and wonder about the enemies of eating.

There are no fat people here in Thailand except for the Anglo-Saxons at my hotel. I feel less wraith-like when I walk down the street. I see the skinny legs and bony shoulders as adaptations, not ruinations. But, still, my neck pokes out of my collar like the straw out of a drink, and my legs look barely strong enough to keep the ground from rising up and crushing me. It's not as bad as it sounds; I mostly handle the feeling by not looking.

"Practice swallowing," the speech therapist said. In English Mandarin—Mandish? Englarin?—she'd say, "Swallow swallow," although I'm not sure if we use periods in English Mandarin or if perhaps we need a comma.

"Gulp be long," I say.

Hypermetaphorosis Sets In

• • •

This is the jogging path in the royal park next to the convention center. At 10:00 a.m., it's got no customers. The woman on the right is wrapped and hatted to keep her skin from tanning. All the models in the cosmetics ads (and there are lots of cosmetic ads here) are white-white.

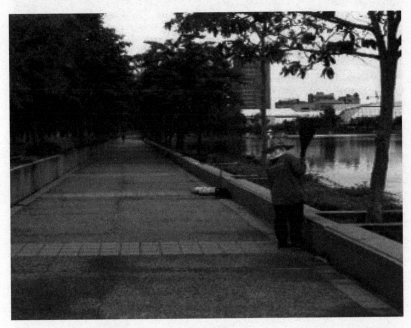

So far, I've resisted the temptation to go for the $219 tailor's special, which includes two custom-made suits, two pairs of pants, two shirts, and two neckties. But I have a few more days here before we go to Saigon . . .

Car traffic is so dense and intense that the city has built walkways over streets, which have then become de facto highways. Cross at your own risk.

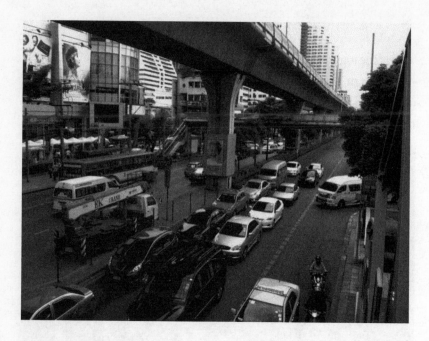

Everybody has something to sell you. The signs on the elevated train say No Hawking, and they ain't talking about falcons. Even the people who work in the hotel want to be your guide after hours, although their offer is "top secret." I send J this poem:

Bangkok Map

I want the knowledge,
I crave the city map, the plan,
the ground with human tracings written small.

The 3rd Assistant Concierge follows me into the garden.
Things have happened in gardens before, I know, my senses serpent-sharp.
I think she said: "Where do you want to go?"
I have no idea where I want to go: hardly ever do
I was hoping this time the map would tell me.
So I stammer something about food and hunger and she says:

Hypermetaphorosis Sets In

"I could show you
good restaurant
good massage
good girl-show. You like girl?
Top secret, don't tell hotel."
"I am lesbian," she goes on. "You don't have to be afraid of me.
I take you to ping-pong show, banana show, cigarette show.
After show, you stay with girl, bring home.
Bring home be good for you, yes?"

I tell her: I can't get much topspin from my paddle:
it makes me resentful of ping-pong,
Cigarettes stink, and
I just had a banana at breakfast. No thanks.

When she walks away, I wonder.
What shows I'd show to go you
if you were here or I were there.
Would I take you to the puppy, kitten, and toddler show?
Or the sashimi and Allagash Tripel show with the Dancing Kumamotos?
Maybe the soulful poetry show with the big chocolate eyes
and the snaky, forearm punctuation?
And after show, would you be my home?
My garden?
My map?
Be good for you, yes?

(Published in the *Baltimore Review*)

The golfers' massage with hot oil is 600 Thai baht (THB), about $25, and the firming massage (lower abdomen) is a mere 1,000 THB, and you can have the Thai traditional for 300. The traditional is a big thing here; there's even a traditional massage school on the royal temple grounds right next to the emerald Buddha.

I get the traditional Thai treatment. You dress in ultra-light cotton pajamas, and a tiny person stretches you, flexes you, and buries her knuckles in your flesh. It's a little like getting beaten up by someone with a plan. After a half hour or so, I drift off into some dream of swimming alongside my own reflection. At the end of the massage, the masseuse has to wake me up, and it is quite a while before I make my way out of the room.

People warned me about eating promiscuously: watch out for the street food, they said. So watch out for it I did. I don't think you could ever get much fresher than this:

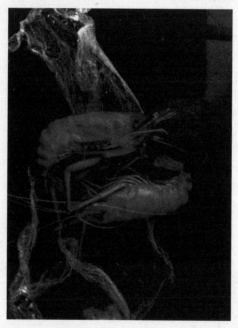

Six-inch (fifteen-centimeter)
prawns at a street restaurant

The steamed food may have salmonella, and the grilled stuff will probably give you cancer. Oh, wait . . .

• • •

Hypermetaphorosis Sets In

One of the reasons I'm in Vietnam is to teach some hospitality students a few things about wine. It's an interesting problem for a few reasons. One of the obvious ones is that this is not a traditional wine-drinking culture. Nobody here has grown up with the romance of wine or its tastes. Even when these students learn to like the taste of wine, they have no idea what wine means to us Westerners. So my approach is a little like a translator's. Here's an excerpt from my handout:

> There's lots to know about wine. Wine has taste; wine has aroma. It has value; it has compatibilities; each wine has an agricultural history and particular storage and handling requirements. We can spend a lifetime learning them. But the person who wants to please his guests and maximize his hospitality business needs to know one very important thing: wine has meaning.

Suspecting how much of their culture I'm completely missing, I will talk about the meaning of tea here in Vietnam. I'm hoping for a little glimmer, hands across the water, stuff like that. Kumbaya.

The other problem is personal. I can no longer taste wine myself. There's nothing wrong with my sense of smell; what's happened is that the radiation killed my salivary glands, so my mouth is typically dry. The tannin in red wine, which usually binds with the salivary protein mucin, instead binds to the Lynn protein of my own personal flesh. Tannin extracts water from protein. In a normal mouth, tannin turns saliva into water, which is washed away by the wine, leaving a dry mouth. (Dry wine dries. Get it?) In my mouth, tannin ignites. It attacks the proteins in my tissues, and it burns. The acid in white wine is a little less painful, but it ain't fun, either. The red wine that I used to drink now drinks me back.

RADIATION DAYS

So here I am, talking passionately about wine. I'm smelling to make sure the stuff is good before I pour for the students. I'm telling them about my passion for the stuff and everything it means to some of their potential guests, and then I say:

> "Wine is well suited to carry all these meanings: at its best, its flavor is complex and intense. It comes in thousands of variations, and its ability to ennoble the taste of most food is near-miraculous. All of the other meanings are built on the taste, and that's what we're here to explore today."

And I can't taste a thing: I'm a deaf musician, a blind photographer. Now you might think that this would leave me depressed or at least sad, and we can both be surprised when I tell you that it doesn't. For one thing, I have wondrous, beautiful beer to console me. (Hey, I could write a book.) For another, I remember that I just escaped across a particularly dangerous burning bridge, and it seems reasonable that there would be a toll. Wine done good by me—no complaints. Better yet, it's even possible that one of these youngsters will leave with a curiosity that grows into an interest that becomes a passion. L'chaim.

After Taste

We met for our tasting yesterday in a tiled echoing room on the Hoa Sen campus. Twelve students, three faculty, and four administrators turned up. A tough crowd.

The way I like to get dialog going is by asking the audience questions, making them part of the show. These folks weren't buying it. It could be limited English skills, maybe cultural reticence. "Has anybody here tasted wine?" No hands. "Anybody here who's never tasted wine?" No hands, either. Anyway, I soldiered through it, and at the end I was mobbed by admirers. And who do you think they were? The administrators. Yup, for the first time in my teaching life, I was more popular with administration than students. Kind of rounds out a career, ya know?

The wines were good. I took micro-sips and did a lot of sniffing. Stars were Tommasi Valpolicella and Ripasso. Antinori Toscana was pretty good, too. Julio and I came back and did the rest of our cooking, then went out in the neighborhood to a fish place with multiple live tanks.

In each one, there's a little salty community of fellows going about their routines, checking each other, swimming forward and backward, grappling for position at the top of the pile, or resignedly contemplating things from the bottom. The tanks would invite comparisons with us except that our taste is not improved by butter.

Here's a picture of the an insect-like critter, maybe thirty centimeters long, that did a pretty good lobster imitation.

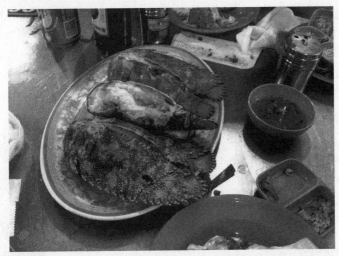

We ate another strange armored creature and a few of the scallops and some gigantic cross between a piss clam and a razor clam (no photo of that one). The bill was $50. In the tradition of first-world visitors to less-developed places, we chuckled at the amount.

The unit is called the Dong, which states the matter rather crudely and makes for some interesting conversation in English.

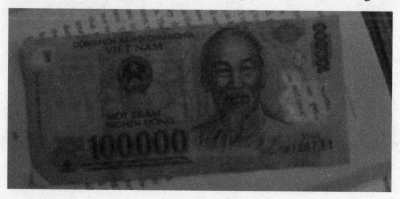

It's rather pretty money: note especially the transparent patches in the upper left and lower right. I like the idea of money you can see through. This bill is worth less than $5. The Dong is so inflated that usual restaurant bills are in the millions. Your typical ATM withdrawal is 2 million VND. I got paid 8 million for my wine tasting. A Vietnamese millionaire.

The portrait is, of course, of Ho Chi Minh. His face is on all the currency. I found it strange, a little alienating, in fact. Even though I was one of those very much against the war, there is no comfort in this image. I had two friends who came back from this war and one who didn't—maybe that's the source of my odd discomfort.

If you're wondering what happened to the Viet Cong:

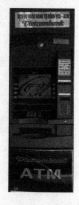

Anyway, the Vietnamese seem to have gotten over it (except for the nasty bit about Agent Orange), so I guess we, or rather I, should, too.

Hypermetaphorosis Sets In

$\bullet\ \bullet\ \bullet$

Just outside of Siem Reap in Southern Cambodia, there is a complex of ruins of Hindu and Buddhist temples. It's collectively called Angkor Wat in the travel industry (a figure of speech referred to as "Schenectady," in which a part is made to stand for an entire small, ruined city). You can speed-walk through the temples in three days, and maybe that's the way to get a sense of the size of this place.

I can vouch for the fact that it's not a good way to get any other sense of it. For one thing, there is a sense of ruin and abandonment about the place that you don't find in other places that have an inheritance like this. You don't leave the temple and skip across six lanes of traffic and grab a nice gelato. You get here at a slog, and the path is dirt, and the fields around seem to be grudgingly bearing crops. The feeling may be a bit unsettling, and that may be why all us tourists become frenetically active here.

Another reason to slow down is that the place is literature as much as it is architecture. The walls and columns are covered, in an encyclopedic, compulsive frenzy, with low relief illustrations of two pieces of classical Indian lit: the Ramayana and the Mahabharata. When I was a kid, there was an exhibit of illustrations from the Ramayana at the New York Public Library (the one with the lions). I remember it mostly as a swashbuckler: demons and monsters and battles. It's also—as my guide explained to me—an intricate description of ideal social life: what it's like to be a soldier, a soldier's wife, a dancer, or a king.

I was lucky to have a translator, but I wasn't smart enough to insist that we take our time and smell the sculpture.

Finally, race-walking encourages you to punctuate your visit with memorials to the picturesque—stop-'n'-snap, stop-'n'-snap.

RADIATION DAYS

What do you remember of Angkor Wat? Taking pictures to catch
your breath, of course. Here are a few of mine:

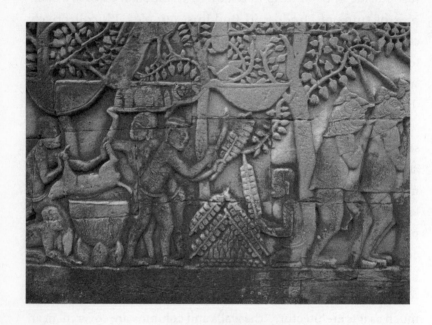

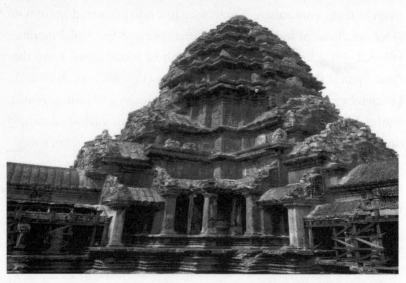

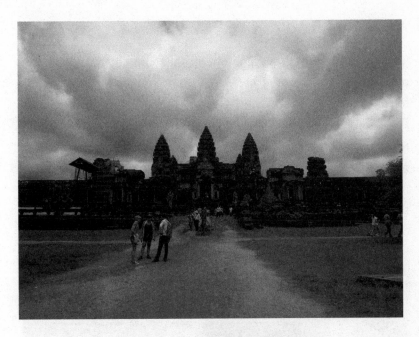

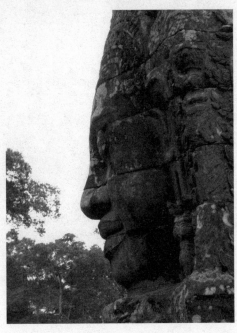

Adolescent Rebellion

There is something about monuments that hangs me in a pendulum cycle from Awe to Boredom. Can't help it. Maybe I'm just not able to stand the sense of Inferiority before the Timeless or maybe, less personally, Awe has its own built-in antibodies. Either way, my photos of monuments are heavy with images of people photographing monuments and images of people photographing other people in monuments. Yes, I understand that this trope is as much a cliché as the pictures of the monuments themselves, but, hey, who am I to argue? So I have another album: a set of pictures of people who—like me—haven't come completely under the spell of the ancient.

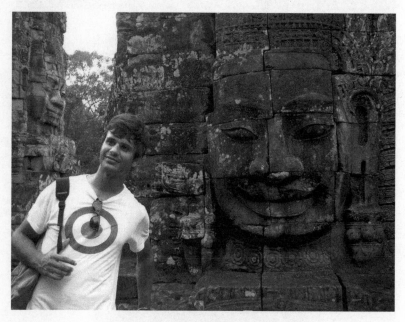

Upright Buddha, leaning tourist.

Hypermetaphorosis Sets In

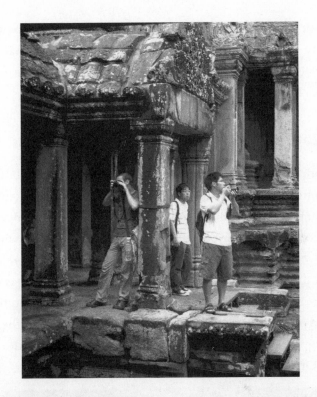

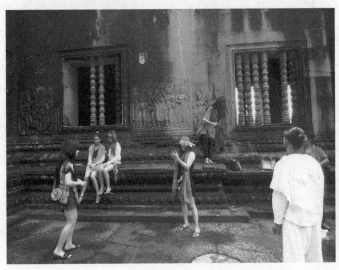

I left with a new appreciation for those places that either ban photography outright or make it grossly impractical by having low light levels. You say you can't take a picture, and all you can do is be there? Exactly.

Flagrant Ingratitude

Every once in a while, as we jogged along, I would see a butterfly. (My friends know that all it takes is one lousy scaly-wing, and my attention flutters off with it—forget Lynn for a while. Penelope Cruz with a cold Allagash Tripel couldn't compete.) My guide, who was both clever and completely professional, picked up on this prejudice.

"Butterflies beat rocks any day," I may have said, which is tough language to use in front of a defender of his people's antiquities.

The photos are terrible, I know. Maybe we can read the blurs charitably, as expressions of my sense of the fleeting nature of all things. Or maybe it's just lousy photography.

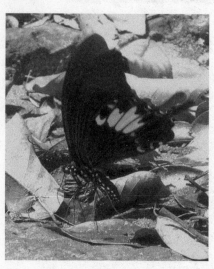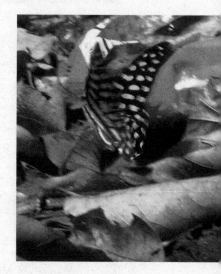

Hypermetaphorosis Sets In

I don't even have a shot of the daisy-yellow creature that landed on my hand. On my hand, fer chrissake! It flew around us for a bit while we were making our way along a shaded path from the road to a temple. It landed on my right hand, and I wondered for a second if I could figure out a way to use the camera with my left and record the moment. I couldn't do it. All I could do was just be there, looking at the slender blackbody with the tiny iridescent green spot behind the head and the pulsing yellow wings.

When I don't have the pictures in front of me, guess what I'll remember about Angkor Wat?

Julio and the Second Thing That Matters

～ I just had this great adventure. I went to Vietnam, I taught a few teachings, learned a few more.

My vanity is still intact, so I'd like you to believe that I got invited on this trip because of my vast knowledge of food and wine and beer and my superior—almost charismatic—skills as a teacher. Even better—maybe it was my subtlety as a chef and exponent of the virtues of Western cuisine that got me imported and important in Saigon. F'r instance, look at this braised oxtail. Wouldn't you invite the guy who could make that to fly halfway 'round the world?

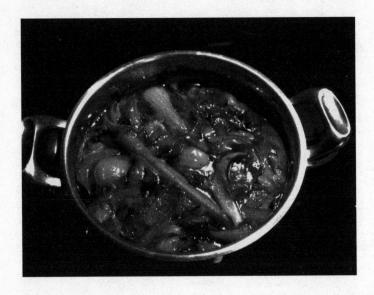

Julio and the Second Thing That Matters

But the truth, dear ones, is that I got this chance for an adventure because of the generosity of a friend. I have, at this late stage in life, only a few friends. (The youngest of them has volunteered to organize my funeral, because he figures it will take just two cars and a case of wine. Fair enough, that's how I've lived it, and, frankly, I'm unlikely to care about attendance at that event anyway.)

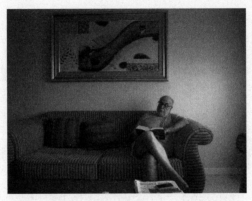

Julio with home furnishings not of his choice.

Julio Aramberri was the department head at a college where I used to teach. He was also head (director general!) of the Spanish National Tourist Office. He writes books in English and Spanish, and thinks heavy cultural stuff for *El Pais* and *La Revista dos Libros*. He is and does all sorts of intellectual heavy lifting. Julio is one of those guys for whom everything in the universe is connected somehow to everything else. As a consequence, no conversation has a necessary conclusion. Even tautologies and imperatives are just introits to the nature of logic and language and nuance and old-ance.

In short, if you have a certain temperament, you'd pay money to hang out with the guy. And yet, by some minor miracle, it's costing him to bring me over to spend time with him. I'm flattered, not in the usual sense of having my own good opinions seconded, but in the rarer sense of being valued in the real-time world by someone I admire, by the smartest guy in the room.

You may sense in that statement the reason that I have only a few close male friends and also why I'm perfectly happy with that small allotment. I know my sense of gratitude doesn't migrate intact from heart to page.

• • •

On my long list of weaknesses, let's fess up to a mild case of Buddha-olatry. I have been charmed, moved, and occasionally made thoughtful by images of the Buddha. My seeking them out isn't so much a matter of looking for spiritual gain as it is a simple matter of enjoying the rush of feelings that sometimes follows a good Buddha viewing. Got my socks knocked off in Kamakura, I did, and I look for a reprise of that thrill, for the same thing but different.

The Reclining Buddha turned out to be the prize puppy of the riverfront temples in Bangkok. Serene and humorous, ready to die, he looks like he's about to tell you a joke. Even the name of the temple—Wat Pho—seems designed to make you smile.

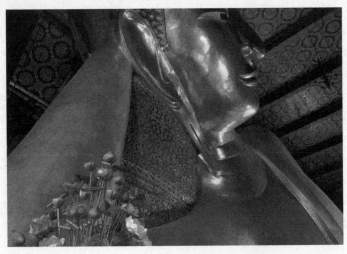

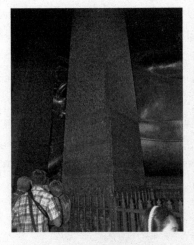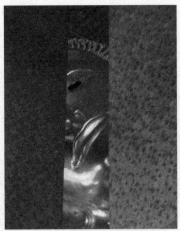

But there's something much more going on here. The statue is huge, forty-six meters long and fifteen high. Half a football field of Buddha entering Nirvana. It's separated from the gallery by a line of columns that make for a peek-a-boo sort of viewing experience.

And then, if the Buddha needs a little help, there's always hydraulic meditation.

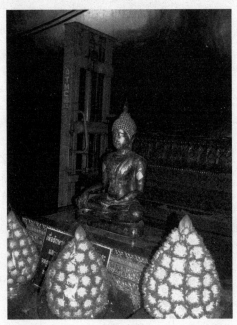

RADIATION DAYS

The Emerald Buddha is just barely visible below in the center left of the window. The statue itself is small, forty-five centimeters (eighteen inches) tall and mostly obscured by its clothing. The strength of the impression comes from the room, which is gilded to a fare-thee-well and decorated with scenes from the life of Buddha. There's also a wonderful Buddha-Nazi attendant who makes sure that everyone is properly respectful. I think I saw a few Euro-Buddhists of the Mahayana persuasions smirking as they hunkered down to meditate, but maybe I'm just projecting that.

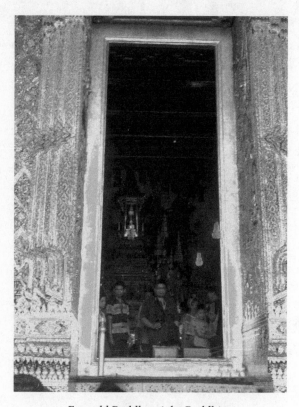

Emerald Buddha, violet Buddhist.

Julio and the Second Thing That Matters

This (from Angkor Wat) is the serenity, the joy that makes these images so appealing to me. It's not the doped-up bliss-face that you see in so much religious imagery; it's something lighthearted and happy.

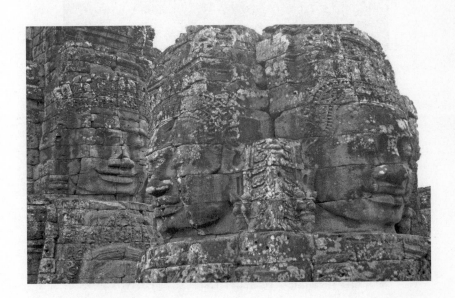

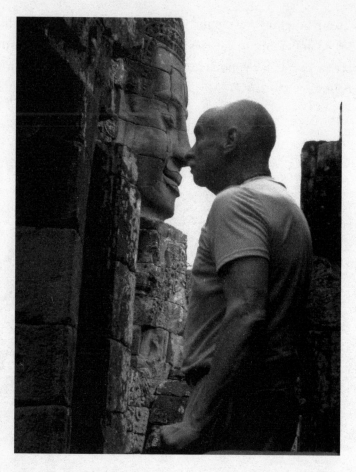

This must be a standard guide prank. The guide takes the tourist's camera and moves him into position, snaps the picture, and laughs. Later the tourist sees himself about to lay a lip lock on the Enlightened One. You have to admit that the Buddha looks as if he likes the idea.

Anyway. On to the Second Thing That Matters. It's generosity, which is related to kindness and is sprinkled with a sense of we're-not-here-forever. My father had it, my daughter shows every sign, and I would pray for it myself if that were the way.

Julio and the Second Thing That Matters

And by way of odd coincidence:

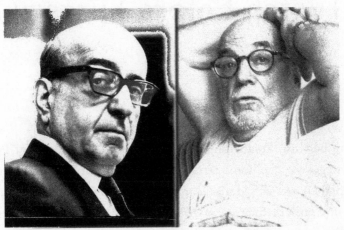

My father, left; Julio Aramberri, right

Wouldn't want to be up against them in doubles at nine-ball, would you?

A Twitch before Surgery

~ I'm back in Philadelphia. In a few minutes, I'll leave for Fox Chase to get the papilloma removed from the floor of my mouth. I feel apprehensive, see clouds, hear hoof beats. So far, I've been pretty steady and present-focused as we have plowed through the process, and today, walking in the woods on a lovely, cool morning, I noticed a touch of—what is that feeling?—I guess it's fear.

Perhaps the feeling is a little bit about the procedure itself (cutting something out of my mouth) and a bit about the recurrence of the lump under my jaw and the shooting pains in the ear. I seem to hear my speech getting thicker and my tongue less agile, too. Maybe I've been denying all this, and today my denial permit is about to expire.

An old friend of mine always advises feeling what you're feeling, so I'll let the fear dance around and see what happens. Stay tuned.

• • •

Here's a rarity for you: a surgeon decided not to operate. Mark the date.

What stayed the scalpel is this: the lump in my jaw and the thickness I'm feeling at the base of my tongue distracted him. Suspicious, he orders an MRI for this Thursday. Could be simply a reaction to the radiation (he tells me that the body keeps on reacting), or it could be a brand-new tumor.

A Twitch before Surgery

When I went to get the date and the follow-up, they gave me Thursday, September 1, for the scan and September 16 for the meeting with the surgeon to discuss the results. Seems a bit cruel, I said. Two weeks wait to find out if it's cancer again?

"Well, the doctor isn't in before that."

"Does he have a fellow? A backup? A pinch-cutter?"

"No."

"What about the oncologist? Or the radiologist?"

"Oh, sir, those are different doctors."

"Yeah, but I'm the same patient."

So the scheduler left her post and went off somewhere. When she came back, I had a follow-up on the sixth, so a week from today, we'll find out what's making a lump in my throat. I don't think it's the compassion of the schedulers at Fox Chase that cut the waiting time in half, so I guess it must be one of two other things. Stay tuned.

Mark Lyons

∼ Walking in the woods this morning, I run into Mark Lyons's dog Cosmo, and a few minutes later I see Mark coming up the hill that Lola and I are descending. Mark is a very sweet, compassionate guy who did me a favor last fall. When the doctors were telling me that I might lose my voice, I asked Mark if he could help me make a recording.

There were some poems that I'd written for my daughter, and I hoped that she would let me read one of them at her wedding. Since it seemed like the chances of my being at this event, much less having a voice to read, were getting pretty slim, I thought it would be nice to record them while I still could and give her a copy. I knew that Mark used voice recording in his teaching, so I asked and he agreed, and as silly as it sounds, the whole thing meant a lot to me.

So I'm always glad to see Mark and Cosmo, and today we stopped and talked about his travels and mine, and when he asked about my health, I told him what I told you yesterday: potential bad moon a-risin', etc. Then I added that otherwise I felt pretty good, and no matter what, there was an excellent chance that I would live to see the World Series. (For those of you from out of town, I should tell you that the Phillies are having a great year anchored by rock-solid pitching and are very likely to be in the fall classic.)

"What?" he said. "How the hell did you get tickets? I'm so fucking jealous! You got Series tickets! I hate you!"

"Um, no, Mark. I'm just glad that there's a good chance that this thing won't kill me before November."

"Oh."

· · ·

Taking an MRI exam is, from the point of view of the slab of meat that's being examined, a lot like taking a PET scan. You're strapped down a bit more, but for us experienced radiation hands, it ain't much. Otherwise, you're slid into a long, coffin-like tube, and you tell yourself that you're not actually buried alive. Then you pay attention to your breaths and give a lot of thought to not moving (which is harder than moving, I tell you).

The only difference is that the MRI machine makes noise. Imagine someone banging on a drum that was filled with scrap metal, and you'll have some sense of it. The soundtrack runs alongside the one you select for your earphones. You don't get lost in the music; it's more like you're cast adrift in a noisy gym where everybody is working out to their own playlist.

Visually, they'll give you a chance to mount a mirror on your head restraint. The angled mirror allows you to look out of the tube, between your feet and into the control room, and also through a second glass to the other MRI room. I recommend the hell out of using the mirror. What it does is give you a view of people in action, but no sound. So it's like looking at an aquarium, the view of which I find very soothing. I watched the two technicians gesturing to each other; I saw water bottles opened and felt my mouth go dry. I watched a woman about my age enter the other room, bent over at the waist and clutching her hospital gown as if it would protect her from something. Was it just modesty? Was she in pain? Was it the last gesture that despair allows you when you're caught in the cancer hospital? Then a third tech, stout and blond, entered the control room and acted out the pantomime of someone doing pushups from a wall. Was she holding back the sea? Repelling Syrian demonstrators? Kneading a roomful of bread? Don't know.

Except for the lack of bubbles, they all could have been little goldfish, one tank behind the other.

I'm sure there's a psychotropic preparation for an MRI like Ativan or bourbon. If I'm unlucky enough to take the exam again, I'm sure my study routine will include one of them. Unfortunately, all I did to get ready was to take a walk a few blocks from J's house. Here's what it looked like:

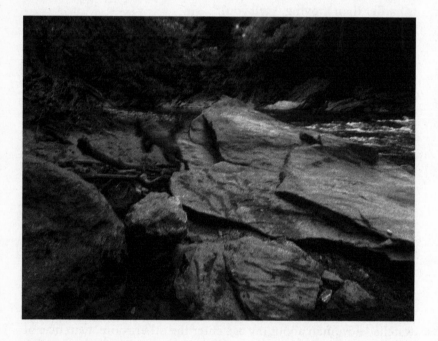

This is right in the city of Philadelphia, and it's just one of hundreds of spots that can get you ready for exams.

Radiation and Relief

∼ The bad news is that it's radiation damage that's messing up my tongue and untrilling my r's. The good news is that it's radiation damage and not a tumor. The radiation damage may get worse; the tumor certainly would get worse.

There's a lot of talk about nerve damage and fibrosis and words like "progressive" and "cumulative." But the distinction gets made between "living with cancer" and "living past cancer," and right now I'm at the beginning of living past it.

How do I feel? I feel like I want to take a nap and write a book and go for a sail and catch a fish and cook it on a little grill on deck and share it with the friends who know the best jokes. I feel like I want to call my dear friend B, who is waiting for her test results, and tell her that there's some good news out in the world and some of it's for her.

I feel like a drink with Gilmore and a dance with J. I feel like swapping recipes and cooking lies. I feel like moving, and when I think about it much, I see a tiny cabin and a boat.

Stay tuned.

Mere Life

〜 It's the meeting with Barbara Burtness, the charming and literate oncologist. I have a book for her: it's *Peace on Earth* by Stanislas Lem. It's a funny book and a little silly. She says that she's coming down with a cold, so we shouldn't shake hands. Nice to worry about colds in the consulting room where we worried about cancer.

There is no evidence of cancer, she says. It begins to sound real, like I hadn't heard it before. There is an effervescence in her voice, and I guess that this is as close as professional decorum lets an oncologist come to the end-zone victory dance. (I would have paid to see her spike a suture kit, wiggle her shoulders, and pound her chest.)

Yeah, I guess a lot of her battles don't end like this, so you probably learn not to over-celebrate the ones that do. Cancer teaches the Middle Way.

So we talk about follow-up and about tending to my radiation damage, and she says goodbye, and we shake hands and then laugh at this terrible breach of prophylaxis. I promise to wash, we laugh again, and then she's gone.

So that's it. After a year, the cancer's gone. Actually, after a year of focusing on cancer, there's nothing left to think about. I'm no longer in the middle of Life-and-Death-Struggle-with-Relentless-Enemy. I'm reduced by a single conversation to mere living. Whatever will I do?

Mere Life

What will I do with the time and the consciousness? What will I do with my blog, for which I have developed some curious feeling of attachment—something like love? Can I abandon it now that the raisin of its *être* is all dried up?

No, of course I can't. At the least, I have to answer the question about what I will do now that I'm reduced to mere living. Gotta justify just being, mere life: what's it all for?

• • •

There are two kinds of answers, a Lesser and a Greater Vehicle. The Lesser answer is that there are a bunch of fun things to pursue, and there's some extra energy to pursue them. I am not at a loss for thoughts about fun.

One pursuit is this poetry obsession. A writing center called Muse House just opened in Chestnut Hill. As near as I can tell, it's the real deal. Actual, accomplished writers with experience in thoughtful coaching and teaching. The poetry teacher is a Kathleen Bonanno. (What will I say to her at New Year's? "Buonanno, Bonanno?" Probably.) Her book—*Slamming Open the Door*—is compact and powerful and dense with truth.

Class starts tomorrow. I'll keep you posted.

• • •

The poetry class turns out better than I thought it could. For one thing, Kathleen, the teacher, is the real deal: a great poet, smart, direct, unflinchingly emotional. For another, she can teach. She reads, sees the bullshit, and calls it out in a gentle way. And there's the matter that I'm the only student—I'm the best damn poet in the class.

The class is for people who've published a little and want to get a book-length manuscript together. My project is called *BOOM!*:

RADIATION DAYS

Poems for a Certain Generation. The method is something like this: first I draw up a map, a story line of everything I've loved for the past twenty years or so. Then I eat some of those neon orange mushrooms that grow in Carpenter's Woods, take off all my clothes, sit in a sweat lodge, and write poems about it all.

OK, I was lying about everything after the part about the map. But the map makes sense. It points to all the emotional termite mounds in the landscape, and that's where the poems seem to be. Beats that ol' Geiger-counter and metal-detector method that I had been using.

Here's one of the first poems from the map. I translated it into Italian because it seemed operatic enough.

note from a libertine, dying

it was not a lack of love
and not, I swear, a love of lacking
love.
it was not a wanting of a better thing
or an eye to the future
or an ear to the past
it was
the flood of you, just you
that washed away the ground
and left me in
a kingdom made of air.

biglietto di un libertino, morendo

non è stata una mancanza d'amore
e non, lo giuro io, l'amore per la mancanza di
amore.
non era un volere di una cosa migliore
o un occhio al futuro
o un orecchio al passato

Mere Life

è stato
il diluvio di voi, proprio voi
che spazzato via la terra
e mi ha lasciato in
un regno fatto d'aria.

(Published in *Philadelphia Poets*)

Mere Life—The Little Stuff—Erotica, et Cetera

~ I always wanted to write a dirty book. The problem was that whenever I got started, about five pages into it, a novel would break out. One of my characters would have a hobby or a crisis or second thoughts. Something outside the bedroom would part the curtains, or something inside the bedroom would swing them shut.

I wrote a sexy book once: it was published under the title *bang BANG*, and now it goes by *Paula Sherman and the National Rifle Association*, but it was really a story about gun crazies and a strong, funny woman who starts a national movement based on the choice between guns and sex. (I hear that someone just won a Nobel Prize for a similar move in Liberia.)

But it wasn't what I wanted. I even got some of the steamy scenes from an unpublished novel called *The Butterfly Farmer* published in a romance magazine, but that didn't do it. I wanted to write about people swept away by desire. I wanted to be in their heads and take the reader in there, too. I wanted to tell sex how much I loved it.

So I finally put together *Philadelphia Personal*. I think I wrote the first grafs about ten or twelve years ago, and I finished it when I was so sick from radiation that I had no sexual feelings of my own. A friend of mine had a contact in the industry and passed it along. It's going to be published in December by the wonderfully named Pink Flamingo Press. They say that if ebook sales are strong, they'll publish actual paper copies. I didn't use a pseudonym; too late for that. If I ever run for president, I'll just say that it was one of those other Lynn Hoffmans who penned this smut.

And so another little item is off the list. Two or three more and then I have to face up to the Big Item, the Greater Vehicle.

In the meantime, my kid ran a half marathon. My darling Spencer, who hated gym and the mandatory teams in high school, pushed and pounded thirteen miles. I cried, of course, but I really don't know why. Why does that sort of intensely solipsistic dedication move us so much? Why do we cheer everybody who slogs across the finish line? Nothing's gained, no one's life is better for it, the sum of human kindness isn't increased, and still we cheer. Sure, there was a charity involved, but I can't remember which one, maybe the Afterthought Foundation.

Oh, and these guys ran, too. Check the sneakers of the fellow on the right.

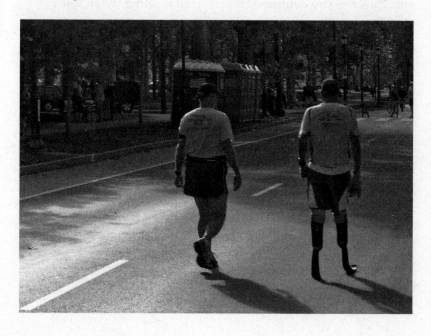

Dis-connected

~ You lose a lot in a divorce—your family, some friends, your home, maybe even your memory, your sense of direction, and your eye for the appropriate. Anyway, I had occasion to write to a friend from those married days about a professional matter. He didn't answer—no real surprise there—but I decided to follow up. It turns out that he's in Sloan-Kettering being treated for leukemia. He's getting chemo, and they're trying to kill him just a little, but not too much, and there he is in the perfect loneliness of dying that somehow ties you compassionately to all us other dying souls.

So here's the feeling: in a flash, I feel connected to him again, and a few minutes later, I find out that my kid knew and never bothered to tell me. Orbital gravity, pulled in, held at a distance: I wonder if there's an equation that describes it, and I hope he has a window with a great view of the city as it whirls around below him.

• • •

That's how my morning started, spitting blood and remembering that this whole adventure got started standing over the same sink. This time, the blood was flowing pretty freely; it hurt a little, and I could feel that it was coming from the site of the surgery about ten days ago.

Dis-connected

A few phone calls and then I was driving myself to Fox Chase with a bloody rag sticking out of my mouth, one hand on the wheel and the other trying to stanch the bleeding. I'm imagining drivers in other cars as they look over at a traffic light and see a guy holding this large red wick in place. Anyway, as luck would have it, it was the WHYY fund drive, a very strange thing to listen to while you're trying not to gag on your own blood. If I hadn't donated just two days before, I would have felt like they were trying to tell me something. I switched stations to WRTI—it's classical music in the morning, and that felt appropriately serious, the sort of soundtrack you'd choose if you were going to pick one for bleeding out in the front seat of your Honda.

(They were playing the overture from *The Merry Widow*, and I'm not married. Go figure.)

An hour later, the bleeding's stopped, and no one has the slightest idea about what may have caused it. I have the feeling that more tests are on the way and I'll see the surgeon again on Friday. Stay tuned.

Acorns

～ The afternoon after they stopped my blood gusher, I went into the woods and planted acorns.

Planting Acorns in Memory of Harold Sills

He's dead you see and
you saved up all your supermarket coupons
and you bought an acre
at the side of the shopping mall and you figure
that you'll never be the sort of soul who puts in an autoparting parlor
or runs a store where people get their nails hammered
and instead of a florist you want a forest
all oaky hokey-dokey
right next to the Home improvement store
for squirrels.
So what you do, see, is to gather the acorns just as they ripen.
And since ripe is dead's first cousin,
you plant the acorns right away and right—
not too far from home. no surprises,
no immigration, no creativity.
you got acorns with filbert worms or weevils?
Feed 'em to the pigs.
wrinkled ones, ones too dry?
throw 'em at your cousin, toss 'em in the sty.
punch holes about as deep as your pinky is long

Acorns

and look at your digit, the planting widget.
go poke for an oak, and leave a tree to grow
a century or three behind you
and every other poky, callused, outdoor jew
and say this prayer
"blessed is the acorn
that blesses me
on the forest floor
for it reminds me to serve the oaks of my children."

In the waiting room now, there's a woman with one of those artificial larynxes and she's talking—in that machine-voiced way—with a woman who's toting a harp. The harp's a pretty, wooden thing about four feet tall, and after some tech talk and pleasantries (Is the wood from pleasant trees? Maybe.) she starts to play, softly giving voice to all of us waiting here for the news from inside ourselves.

And then there's this:

planting acorns—fairmount park

the pain came back, big, dull, personal.
it returned to the old neighborhood
and moved in next door to
where it used to live.

he recognized the pain, of course
and of course, he had forgotten
all about it.

the tests showed what
the shows always test:
that the patient don't have long to wait

RADIATION DAYS

and that he could believe
but in the end, the end
was written with the beginning.

he gathered acorns from the sidewalk
and the road and the beds of his neighbors'
pick-up trucks. he filled a bag with
a brown, promiscuous mix, two pounds, three.
dense, heavy, damp.
he sawed the straw-end off a broomstick
and went to the woods, poking and planting
each acorn on its side two inches down
gravely safe and covered in forest dirt.
he spread the empty bag on a spongy stump
and sat and looked along the way he'd come
and imagined first the dusting then the full sudsy
slather of the coming white concealing snow.

(Published in *The Cancer Poetry Project*)

Nothing to It

～ The surgeon speaks as he walks into the room: it's just a wart, he says. Aside from the disgusting aspect of having had a wart inside your mouth (Will anyone ever kiss me again? Anyone who's read this?), it's a relief. What about the blood gusher? Well, the surgeon's joke is that all bleeding stops eventually, and this bleeding did, too. So what was I worried about? See you in three months.

Of all the relationships in your life, the one whose diminishment you can most fondly endorse is the one with your surgeon. Nice guy and all, maybe even an intellect worth your wiles, but frankly it's best to stop meeting like this, and three months sounds pretty good.

Three months is a season. Nice chunka change. End of summer into winter here in Philadelphia. Last tomatoes into ice-topped ponds. Time to do stuff. A season of writing and life-arranging, paring down if not pairing off. Time for all the Lesser Vehicle things, ticking off stuff I always wanted to get done. Then, if there's a next season, on to the Greater Vehicle.

I Wish

∼ There are some things, some accomplishments that I can only admire humbly from a distance. No chance that they will ever be on my list or that their completion will be nominated here. I don't mean pie-in-the-sky stuff like a Nobel Prize or meeting Terry Gross; I mean things whose beauty and elegance are within my reach. From today's *Times*, in a story about Theo Epstein leaving the Red Sox to take a job with the Cubs:

> *Epstein left the team once before, in 2005, fleeing Fenway Park in a gorilla suit on Halloween after a tiff over his contract extension went public.*

I can hardly imagine having a contract, let alone a contract extension, but "fleeing Fenway Park in a gorilla suit"? Ah, that's the stuff of dreams.

Speech Therapy

～ Radiation does sloppy work. It's not like a good union electrician, let's say, who wipes his fingerprints off the switch plate and sweeps up the flecks of plaster and bits of plastic insulation when the job is done. Therapeutic radiation is more like the fireman, smashing down doors and leaving puddles where your couch used to be.

One of the things it left behind on my tongue is fibrosis—scars to you and me. The scars are stiff and inelastic, and they take the place of the dead muscle. So, the tongue that used to trip lightly along a lecture or a dirty joke or a sonnet is now kind of heavy, stumbling when it trips. I can hear my speech becoming thick and dull. The effect is worse in Italian than English and worst when two consonants sound right next to each other. Other people ask me to repeat myself, and sometimes the sound of my own voice makes me wonder who's talking.

So, now I'm getting speech therapy. The strategy is to build up the muscle in my tongue until I can crack walnuts with it and to simultaneously increase its flexibility. Lingual yoga and isometrics all conducted in the private gymnasium of my very own mouth.

I met with the therapist a few days ago, and we have a date for this week. I stick my tongue out at her a lot, and sometimes I read poems in English and Italian. A little bit of Hoffman, a little bit of Montale. It all seems oddly invasive, as if I were discovering a sense of modesty I didn't know I had. Ashley—my therapist—did teach me one great trick: you can replace the trilled "r" of Italian (impossible to say with a fibrotic tongue) with a "d" spoken quickly. It wouldn't let you pass as a Roman, but in most other places, it would be just fine.

In the meantime, I'm sitting at a traffic light sticking my tongue out and down, holding for five seconds, then stretching it out and up as high as it will go. I don't know if this will improve my speaking voice at all, but it's bound to start some interesting conversations.

• • •

For several days, I had been pacing with a typescript in hand, reading slowly and overenunciating some poems that I had planned to read at Musehouse on Friday. It was a group reading, and my mentor there asked me to join the group.

There were about ten readers. (Do I dare call us poets?) Five men, middle-aged and up, and five women, early twenties and down. The men read about loss and mortality and doubts; the women read about love and family and the excitement of finding a self. Better yet, two friends showed up just to give me some friendly faces to address.

Two surprises: I got through the poems without much trouble, although the enforced slowness may have changed the message a bit; it was kind of fun to leave my Brooklyn pace behind and pretend I was a Mississippi Yankee for a change.

The other surprise was what good entertainment it turned out to be. The ideas were provocative and the readers very personable. Compared to most nights at the theater or music venue, it was comfortable, congenial, and free.

Today, I see that another poem has been published; it's about getting well in the modern world. I find myself wondering what that

Speech Therapy

poem would have sounded like if I weren't one of the lucky ones with private insurance.

The Ballad of Health Care, by the Republican Senators of the United States—*Musical Accompaniment on the Penny Whistle*

Little Marie has outgrown the braces
That allow her to walk and to play
There's no insurance for little Marie:
The dumb little kid was just born that way

Hey diddle your dee and whoop Dee doo
We're Republican senators all
Perhaps her church and the Tea Party Gang,
Will catch her if she should fall.

Tony's kidneys gave up the ghost
And his dialysis credit did too
Tony'll probably be dead in a week
Aren't you glad that he isn't you?

Keisha's meds cost a thousand a month
And she makes just a grand and a half
Could we lower the prices and give her a break?
We could, but don't make us laugh.

Jose got a cut while harvesting grapes
And he's now filled with fever and pus
We'll see him deported if he doesn't die first
We're so happy that he isn't us!

Way out here in our dark red states
We all hate the government doles
Except for the millions in farm subsidies

RADIATION DAYS

Which keep us in health at the polls
Hey diddle my middle and fa-la screw you
We're Republican senators all
Our friends in insurance are as pleased as can be
We know they'll remember next fall.

So bend yourself over and take a deep breath
We're about to give you the wood
And then we'll convince you that we're your best friends
And it's all for your very own good.

We've taken good care of the rich and the strong
We've done everything that we could
And now we'll convince you that we're your best friends
And it's all for your very own good.

(Published in *New Verse News*, *Chestnut Hill Local*, and *Healthy Artists*)

Hard to Believe

〜 Yesterday, around dinner time, I realized that the day had slipped past me—lived in a fog of ordinariness, as if I had all the time in the world. The magic feeling of radiation days had slipped away.

So, this morning, I walked very slowly in the woods, off the trail, spent extra time petting the dog, talking to the naturalist who showed me where to look for the winter wrens. You can only count on cancer to keep you alive for a while, and when the magic wears off, you gotta do it yourself.

• • •

I won't tell you much about Jeff Smith, but I'll tell you that he is the keeper of memories, the soul of kindness, a beatnik, a jazz buff, a man who's been to war. He remembers where he was when Kerouac died and where I was when he called me to tell me about it. He remembers visiting my widowed father and riding the subway home to keep him company. He remembers what it was like to be crazy just for fun, and he knows that the times got sober, so he got saner with them.

We had dinner in Miami Beach tonight, at some little jazz club on Lincoln. He's taking care of his sweetheart, wondering about his friends. He lives in a tiny flat in an old building on the beach. He asks about my daughter, my dog, my woods, my worries. He's totally there, and he says that he thought he'd never see me again, and, damn, ain't it great? And he says it, not so's I'll agree with him, but so he can be sure that I'll feel it myself.

Tomorrow is Thanksgiving. I'll be giving thanks. Hey, it would be crazy not to.

• • •

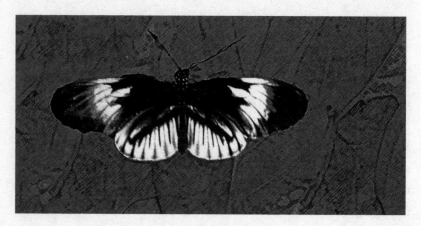

Heliconia

You know those heartwarming stories about somebody who's looking at death and gets a wish and wants to live to see the next Super Bowl, and then some rich guy stakes him to a ticket, and sometime later, March or April, let's say, you hear that the poor bastard croaked, and the guy with the slick hair on the local news says, "Well, at least he got to see the Packers beat the Steelers," and you try not to throw your shoe at the flat screen because, after all, these things cost money?

You do? Good.

Because here's a similar story: guy's withering away from cancer and cancer meds, and he looks sort of like a Peking duck without the shellac, and while he's sad about missing the World Series, what he thinks about in those minutes before the painkillers kick in is that he'll never get back to Butterfly World with its big, floppy tropical butterflies pupating and copulating and flopping around in the dappled sunlight, and frankly butterflies always made him happy, so not seeing them ever again makes him sad as a stand-in for all the sadness of leaving the party while there's still some nectar around, and then the son-of-a-bitch doesn't die, and he puts on a few pounds, and there he is under the netted tent, and there's a half-dozen owl butterflies *manging* on brown bananas, and a malachite lands on his hat, and the woman he's with turns away, because at least he got to see butterflies again, and you know how grown men can be affected by *Lepidoptera*.

Oh. And there was a day in the Everglades, too.

Speaking of *Lepidoptera*

➰ I wrote a poem a while back called "The Would-Be Lepidopterist" about a guy who might have made something out of himself (as if his self weren't something already) if he hadn't been... well, himself. It was published in this beautiful journal called *Off the Coast*, a literary review from Maine.

I just found out that *Off the Coast* used one of its five Pushcart Prize nominations on "Lepidopterist." Getting a Pushcart nomination is sort of like getting an associate's degree or getting promoted to buck sergeant, maybe like turning your learner's permit in for a grown-up license. If you weren't sure before, you can now at least say that you're a poet and keep a straight face. (Although why you'd want to either say that or keep from giggling about it is beyond me right now.)

Anyway.

Here's the poem again:

The Would-Be Lepidopterist

You would have known more about butterflies
if you had killed them more and watched them less.
If you had used a killing jar and a scalpel and collected
the various, variegated genitalia
of Nymphs and Satyrs, Blues and Coppers.
You could have been.

Speaking of Lepidoptera

But no, you only planted flowers for them to suck
and sheltered the weeds where they laid their eggs
And applauded when you saw them jump into the air
and wink their way along their next performance.
Applauded! (Who the hell were you applauding?)

No eternity for those bugs or you,
Just a messy, scaly, insect stew.
No dry forever on a pin,
Just vanished scale on a dusty wing.

So you don't know much about butterflies,
You even forget their names from time to time.
You can't tell a Painted Lady from an American,
Vanessa cardui from Vanessa whaz-er-name.

All you have left is that stupid, sharp indrawn breath
as you see the Mourning Cloak
(arrogant first-bastard of spring)
spread her wings and pump the April into them
to mark the end of March.

You would have known more about so many things
if you hadn't whooped and danced and shook your fists
as the chrysalis broke and gold wet wings appeared.

(Published in *Off the Coast*)

Note on an Unlikely Birthday

Happy Birthday

The old man's muscles, vines
grown tight around a wrinkled trunk,

they're warning of a smaller crop,
promising richer, darker fruit.
Having fun? he said.
   Well, I . . .
Fun is good, he said.
It's medicine against romantics, he said.
The romantics are like the shingles
or the vine louse, he said,
they hurt like hell, they kill the root.
You caught a cold,
you need the cure, he said.
Have fun.
   Do I know you?
You will, he said.
Happy Birthday

• • •

I know that there's some bigger thing for me to do with the extra time that I've been given, and I'm chasing that thing down, tracking it in the forest maybe. It's hard for me to see, the woods being dark and all and so many ego-bright creative desires in my eyes. But I'm chasing it: I know it has to do with teaching or tending a garden, and I won't stop looking.

In the meantime, there's art. Or maybe "art." Anyway, there are things I've always wanted to write and do. One of them is an erotic novel. I've written a few lascivious things before, little pieces, poems, the occasional love note, but I've always wanted to stare at the thing itself without getting dizzy. Just for fun, ya know.

Next? There's a chapbook that's been accepted, and the *Short Course in Beer* that's scheduled for May. While I'm waiting, I'm flogging a volume of poems called *BOOM!: Poems for a Certain Generation* and looking at a novel about love and longing in South Philly. I'm also

Speaking of Lepidoptera

reviving my picture lust, thinking that in the absence of a physical studio, I'll learn some digital techniques and play with that.

I know I should be saving the world, but this sure is fun. There's something I want to say to everyone who's dealing with cancer or one of its buddies right now: Screw "hope." Forget it. Hope's a thief; it steals your life. You don't want hope, or Hope—you want to live right now.

There's Hope

Hope snaps a polished metal bowl
around your neck. He collars you
like a pair o' bollocks. You can bathe
in the starlight, reflected, focused, magnified.
Your glance is forever up,
Hope appoints you
to heaven, to galaxies that hold all
the archers, gods, and possibilities.
Of course, you can't see yourself,
you can't look down, or out
(Hope will not allow it)
and you'll miss *Papillio glaucus*
bouncing on the milkweed.
Dear Hope insists that you never see the snake
or smell the grass.
And the sun of mid-day,
(Hope's favorite time) will focus
on your head and boil your brain,
the steam from which—
please note—will rise up
in broad, expanding surges to the sky.
Or so he Hopes.

(Published in *Musehouse Journal*)

RADIATION DAYS

• • •

Forgive me—it's time to turn to other things: less dramatic, more like life than life and death.

Last night at dinner, I had a glass of red wine. An Aglianico called Rocca del Dragone from the Greek part of southern Italy, ripe and round like lust or a good old joke. It only hurt a little, and it was delicious. I can't say that my old friend is back, but if I need something for a sacrament, I think I can go to the red again.

I feel a moral coming on—maybe two morals.

One is that when you're sick, don't give in to Hope. Hope is bullshit. Take charge, get good help, do the best you can to recover, but don't waste your time with Hope. Instead, spend your time in the here and now. Make that Here and Now. Live each day, and if you're deathly sick, steal some little fragment of life: the butterflies, the walk in woods, the smell of oregano or babies, a visit from Nyheim or Gilmore, a minute with J or your kid.

The other is that when you're well, drench yourself with memories of present beauty; put that stuff in the bank. Make pictures, get painted, make recordings of voices and songs, write by hand on the back of menus, keep baby books for your kids and love notes for yourself. Oh, yeah, and spread the joy around.

And, by the way, the reward of a good attitude isn't good health. The reward for having a good attitude is that you get to enjoy your life.

Now.

Speaking of Lepidoptera

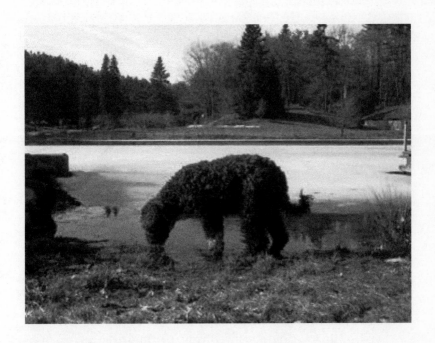